Rapid Weight Loss Hypnosis and Meditation

The Complete Guided to Lose Weight. Stop Overeating, Reduce Eating, Healthy Habits, Exercise Motivation, Deep Sleep and more with Self-Hypnosis & Meditation

Claire Heng

Disclaimer Notice:

Please note the information contained within this document is for educational and entertainment purposes only. All effort has been executed to present accurate, up to date, and reliable, complete information. No warranties of any kind are declared or implied. Readers acknowledge that the author is not engaging in the rendering of legal, financial, medical, or professional advice. The content within this book has been derived from various sources. Please consult a licensed professional before attempting any techniques outlined in this book.

By reading this document, the reader agrees that under no circumstances is the author responsible for any losses, direct or indirect, which are incurred as a result of the use of the information contained within this document, including, but not limited to, — errors, omissions, or inaccuracies.

Table of Contents

Introduction

I need to begin by congratulating you on getting this guide - ***Rapid Weight Loss Hypnosis and Meditation for Women***.

There is no denying that obesity and, therefore, the associated health problems are among the most critical challenges faced not only by western countries but also in many other developing countries. The Journal of Health Economics provides quite $ 200 billion annually within us for medical obesity research costs. Consistent with SAD (Standard American Diet), processed foods and beverages high in fat, sodium, and sugar spread to other countries, increasing heart condition, diabetes, and other life-threatening problems. The food industry has been treating overweight people for many years - most of the people have tried various diets and other programs that either fail or work temporarily and have made them even more discouraged.

You will find plenty of help books that offer you diet plans, but they're useless. If you question this, when trying to satisfy the diet's requirements, including allowing all of the ingredients, you'll reduce with only the trouble required to follow the diet. But here is that the most crucial statistic that anyone who wants to reduce should know. Most of the people who reduce successfully continue a diet and gain even more weight within the first year! These statistics include people that have participated within the Biggest Loser or whose stomachs are stapled. This way is often the foremost suppressed statistic within the food industry: only 3 in 100 people that reach their goal manage to take care of this weight loss beyond the first year.

A post-mortem with the remainder of the 97 people that struggled to stay their burden showed that they were much hungry after trying their regular diet again than they were before the load loss program. They need been busy eating since the top of their diet, and a few are crazy about food.

From the attitude of human evolution, eating is that the phenomenon of the last second. Historically telling, the 1920s was a mere failure to market less eating, but as a society, the cycle of dietary habits that triggered famine brain mechanisms began until the late 1960s.

A weight-loss diet, by definition, requires a discount in food intake below what the body must maintain its current form. There's no real food shortage, but all the built-in mechanisms that ensure our survival record fat loss. This reduction triggers a neural circuit that uses a military of hormones that cause the order of overeating. This mechanism is just called the famine brain.

Overeating works because of the brain's primary reward system for dieting. Unfortunately, researchers have found that weight loss of all types uses our neurochemical weapons. If you've got an excessive amount of fat, your body won't know. It only "knows" if you risk losing fat. During a bold plan to regain homeostasis, our system lowers the hormone levels that signal satiety (leptin and insulin) and pumps the fasting hormone 'ghrelin' into the bloodstream. This hormone leads to heightened looking for food resulting in extra calorie intake and eventually more weight gain.

Scientists aren't yet conscious of how the brain and physical starvation system interact to support or override one another. What we all know is that a lot of regular diets cause a mind hooked into food. Therefore, the basis of the matter lies within the brain, where this cycle continues.

The way we will save us from this cycle is to optimize brain activity. This optimization and control are what you'll learn during this book.

Thankfully, we will change our brain patterns to behave differently. During this book, we'll study self-hypnosis, cognitive behavioral therapy, sleep learning system, and meditation to regulate our brain and overcome food cravings. To quickly put, we'll optimize brain activity.

It also covers seemingly ordinary but very influential tricks to urge and prevent excess fat. We'll also learn a couple of practical habits employing the techniques mentioned above. We'll investigate the situation of the matter and the way it affects us so that we will suggest targeted actions.

Understanding Hypnosis

When you believe hypnosis, you'll consider a mysterious person who would swing a watch before your eyes. Afterward, you'll probably think that a person who falls under hypnosis would do anything that the hypnotist orders him as if they need suddenly created a master-slave relationship in a moment. However, this therapy runs more profound than that of popular culture belief.

By Definition

Hypnosis is that the technique that permits you to travel into that state of your consciousness wherein you allow a part of your brain responsible for your subconscious to dominate your thought process. Meaning that once you are being hypnotized, you tap the proper hemisphere of your mind, which is responsible for your automatic actions, creativity, and imagination.

Hypnosis also causes you to very vulnerable to suggestions and influence. Since you're suppressing a part of your brain that dictates logic, you're ready to suspend your current beliefs about what you'll do. That permits this system to form suggestions, make your mind allow suppressed memories to resurface, or maybe assist you change your behavior.

Hypnosis has been a really controversial technique – because it can make an individual consider things that he would usually wouldn't, to the purpose that it can lead an individual to perform something that appears to be outside his will, some view this system to be dangerous.

However, a deeper understanding of what happens during hypnosis will cause you to see what may happen under a trance and up to what point can an individual be commanded under therapy. Within the end, you'd even have a far better understanding of how an individual's mind is often manipulated.

What Happens Once You Are Hypnotized?

Whenever you enter a trance, you'd describe the sensation to be very almost like what you experience once you are daydreaming. You'll imagine things that you only usually cannot, an equivalent as what your mind triggers while you're within the state of a dream when sleeping. You'll imagine yourself flying, doing the critical Superman punch, and so on, but the thing is, you're awake and hyper-attentive.

Why do people think that once you are hypnotized, you're actually during a sleep state? The rationale is that once you are focusing intensely on anything that you simply want to indeed concentrate on, you lose yourself. It's almost like watching a movie or reading a book – you feel that all scenarios may happen in the real world, and your emotions are engaged.

You suspend your beliefs for a flash then enjoy the chances that are presented to you. Almost like reading a book or watching a movie, it's up to you to believe if what you're watching or reading can happen in the real world. Meaning that you simply have complete discretion to think or do anything under hypnosis – you'll choose whether you would like to resist an order or a suggestion that's offered to you. If you select not to participate with the hypnosis, then there's nothing that a hypnotist can do to form you are doing an action or consider an idea.

Why does this happen? Whenever you permit access to your subconscious during a hypnosis session, you'll feel that you simply are during a state of relaxation, but you're genuinely awake. Because you're allowing yourself to surrender to your imagination, your subconscious begins to figure behind the scenes and project images and scenarios in your mind. However, your conscious mind remains actively participating in your thoughts, and you'll still know that a number of the items that you simply see wouldn't be possible in the real world. However, your subconscious would even allow you to form the use of your emotions.

Once your emotions are triggered within the event that your subconscious projects inside your mind, you'd be ready to formulate ideas using your conscious mind. This way causes you to feel inspired or have a specific concept you'll execute while you're fully awake.

Similar to daydreaming, hypnosis can trigger inspiration supported ideas that are planted during a script that you simply read otherwise you heard.

After a hypnosis session, you'll suddenly have that urge to try something that you simply wouldn't believe doing within the past. When that happens, you're working on the suggestion that you simply heard or saw, but it's still up to you to offer into. Since you're highly suggestible under a trance, you'll find it difficult to disregard that thought, as if your brain has been re-programmed during a particular manner.

Why Learn or Experience Hypnosis?

You can hypnotize yourself – all you would like to try to is to read a hypnosis script or hear a hypnosis audio track to induce yourself into a trance and make use of the suggestions that you want to adapt.

Most people welcome the thought of foundering hypnosis or find out how to try to it themselves due to the following reasons:

- It helps them do things that they usually prevent themselves from doing.

Everyone struggles with a selected behavior, and everybody wants to possess control over their actions and beliefs, especially those that are preventing them from meeting their goals. Some people are aware that their fears are preventing them from discovering their potentials.

Some people also are handling bad habits that they feel they can't remove from their routine. To possess power over automatic behaviors, they might get to welcome the likelihood that they're actually on top of things.

- It helps them deal with pain and manage stress and anxiety.

Most of the time, the old saying "mind over matter" is correct. If your mind tells you that your back seems like it's been hit by a sledgehammer, then your body would feel that way. An equivalent happens once you are experiencing extreme stress and anxiety – if you're compelled to think that you cannot deal with your pressures, then your behavior will adapt to the present thought. However, if you become ready to switch your brain into thinking otherwise, then you'd be prepared to allow yourself to feel better.

- It allows you to trigger your confidence.

Some people think that they're too shy and daunted by people around them, to the purpose that they believe they can't do anything right when people are watching. If you think that that is applicable to you, then you'll use hypnosis to assist you in bringing out your hidden confidence.

- It helps you discover ways to be more efficient.

Their routine hinders some people to such extent that they'll believe that they cannot discover a more creative and efficient way of doing things. By allowing some people to renew themselves, they will adopt more productive habits that might enable them to realize their goals in no time in the least.

- It helps you to speak better and influence people.

Learning how to hypnotize people by using techniques that you can easily use in your lifestyle would allow you to tap into the consciousness of others. This way can assist you in putting ideas across and influencing people, even people who seem to possess daunting barriers around them. By learning the way to communicate better and make use of suggestions, you're opening up opportunities that are impossible for you to tap into the past.

These are just some of the items you simply would enjoy once you discover how to hypnotize and become hypnotized. Now, it is time for you to find out the Self Hypnosis technique.

Self-Hypnosis

Self-hypnosis features a powerful ability to assist you in accomplishing virtually anything you desire to realize. Whether you would like to scale back or manage stress, motivate yourself to achieve something, relax from pressure, or other upsetting emotions, Self-hypnosis will assist you. It'll help you to concentrate more efficiently or effectively on a task at hand, or direct yourself to try to or accomplish something; self-hypnosis can assist you drastically.

How Does One Enter A Hypnotic State?

When it involves effectively making use of self-hypnosis, it's generally crucial that an individual has first experienced hypnosis in another form. This way will include attending knowledgeable hypnotherapist and being hypnotized, or it's going to incorporate regular practice through guided hypnosis sessions which will be retrieved through audio files. A private first must learn to become conversant in the hypnotic state and what it seems like before embarking on self-hypnosis, as this may make sure that they're clear on what to look for and what to expect. While you'll undoubtedly engage in self-hypnosis without prior experience or practice, this might reduce results and benefits as you'll not be clear on what to expect or how the training or process should be facilitated.

Once you've experienced some hypnosis, you ought to have a reasonably good idea of what expect and what is going to be achieved during the practice. You'll be conversant in how the hypnotic state is made, what it seems like, and what happens once you've got entered a hypnotic state. From there, you'll follow these same practices to realize the hypnotic state in your self-hypnosis practice.

The hypnotic state isn't guided by an external influence when it involves self-hypnosis. Instead, it is achieved through facilitating deep relaxation within yourself and your body. You are doing this through a series of breathing practices and intentions, whereby you clear your mind and focus solely on your body and breath. This way is often very almost like meditation practice, so people that are already fluent in achieving a relaxed state through meditation will have a general idea of how self-hypnosis is usually made. If you've got not practiced meditation within the past, it's going to be ideal to start your practice now so that you'll practice entering a deep state of relaxation that permits your mind to be influenced by hypnosis.

How Are You Guided?

When it involves self-hypnosis, you're guided by yourself. This way comes through self-suggestion, also as self-exploration. The simplest thanks to guiding yourself through an intentional hypnosis practice are to line the expectation of what you would like to be guided through or toward before you enter the hypnotic state. For instance, say that you simply want to hypnotize yourself and practice self-hypnosis as a way to assist you in quitting something, like smoking. Before entering the state of deep relaxation that's required for hypnosis, you'd set this intention and repeat it to yourself and over and over. Then, you'd begin performing on setting yourself into the hypnotic state of deep relaxation. Once you therein state, you'll start repeating the intention over and over once more. This way may fix the purpose into your mind and permit the message to sink even deeper into your subconscious, allowing it to assist rewrite and re-program your subconscious even as the other form or state of hypnosis would.

Being during a state of both physical and mental deep relaxation like that which is experienced once you are undergoing hypnosis means the intention you set. Therefore the message you repeat goes far beyond your conscious mind. Your conscious mind is that the "first step" of your brain that's wont to process information. This a part of your brain will readily attest or contest anything that you feed your brain with. The thought is to permit yourself to enter a deep state of relaxation. Then you direct your mind through intention. These intentions bypass your conscious mind into the subconscious, which is liable for all that you simply do. This way leads to information which will not be serving you being redesigned by your intention, making it easier for you to facilitate complete changes.

How is Anything Achieved Through This?

The ability to realize results through self-hypnosis works an equivalent as your ability to achieve results through any hypnosis. Whether we know it or not, our subconscious or unconscious is directly liable for virtually everything that we do. This way is often where our "survival" information is stored. Anything that urges us to leap into action or produce specific results are all stored within this a part of our mind and is liable for virtually everything that we do. From breathing and digesting food that we eat to telling us who to trust and who do not, and even helping us make an opinion about things and form judgments on various topics, our subconscious is directly liable for these actions.

The conscious mind can recognize and become aware of things, but it's indirectly liable for what we ultimately prefer to do. So, by consciously choosing to form a change, we must then relay that become our subconscious so that it happens. Even as with the other sort of hypnosis, performing self-hypnosis allows you to require a conscious desire to vary and relay it back to your subconscious so that it takes effect, and actual changes are seen and experienced in our lives. For instance, if you would like to prevent biting your nails, you'll tell you're conscious mind that you simply want to try to so. Then, later, you start biting your nails without realizing it because it's a practice that has become a neighborhood of your subconscious psyche. Therefore, if you would like to instill real change, you've got to bypass your conscious mind and directly tell your subconscious to vary this behavior. This way is often achieved through self-hypnosis, and therefore the results are often as powerful as the other sort of hypnosis.

Regular Hypnosis vs. Self-hypnosis

There truly is not any major difference between regular hypnosis and self-hypnosis, apart from who is facilitating the hypnotic state and directing the subconscious therein state. Regular hypnosis is facilitated by a third-party to address the connection between your conscious and unconscious while self-hypnosis, on the opposite hand, however, is completed directly between your conscious and unconscious and allows you to perform the practice at any given time, in any given place, for any particular reason.

Choosing between self-hypnosis and hypnosis is personal, and both have their unique benefits that outweigh the advantages given by the opposite. For instance, if you're inexperienced and are looking to be hypnotized by knowledgeable to realize something big like to motivate yourself to reduce or become healthier, professional hypnosis can assist you in facilitating this alteration. Professional hypnosis is going to be ready to facilitate quicker results than an inexperienced self-hypnosis practitioner, and that they also will be prepared to use a broader range of words and intentions because they're not within the hypnotic state. Still, rather you're, and that they are simply directing it. By this understanding, a hypnotherapist can take you thru a broader range of intentions and experiences when it involves hypnosis.

However, professional hypnotherapists can become rather costly and should not always be ready to provide you the extent of help that you simply need for various intentions. For instance, they'll not entirely understand what change you would like to form, they'll not be within your budget, or they'll simply not be available at the precise times that you simply need hypnosis to assist you. In these cases, self-hypnosis may be a great option. You'll enter a hypnotic state, then specialize in your intention and, as a result, facilitate change directly at the instant that change is required. This way will increase the advantages and effects you experience from your hypnosis, and it can make hypnotherapy simpler for you.

If you're wondering which to settle on, hypnosis with knowledgeable hypnotherapist or self-hypnosis, the simplest answer is to settle on both. Seeking help from knowledgeable hypnotherapist can assist you to study hypnosis and start navigating the planet of hypnotherapy during a shorter amount of your time. Then, coupling this practice with a self-hypnosis practice can assist you in getting the foremost out of your experience and seeing greater results. You'll engage in shorter, more direct self-hypnotherapy sessions as required to supplement your professional hypnotherapist's findings and ultimately facilitate a complete change.

As you become more practiced with self-hypnosis, you'll begin to get that you do not need the maximum amount of help from professional hypnotherapists. While seeking professional aid within the face of major, difficult, or stubborn changes could also be desirable, you'll likely find that you can facilitate significant changes during a shorter time, the more you practice. For that reason, you become your change-maker and influencer. This way will make the thought of accelerating your skills around self-hypnosis more desirable. It may prove why it's essential to start practicing and taking advantage of this incredible practice as soon as possible.

Conditions for Hypnosis to Figure Out

Although hypnosis itself can't be accurately predicted, clinical experience and laboratory experiments at institutions like Harvard and Stanford suggest that those that are most vulnerable to hypnosis tend to share specific characteristics. As already mentioned, virtually everyone can enjoy hypnosis. However, if you've got most of those characteristics, studies have shown that you simply could also be easier to hypnotize than others. Here are a number of the standards for hypnosis:

- **Motivation**

The motivation is at the highest of the list. If you do not want to be hypnotized, you won't. If you're strong enough to vary something, the prospect is to be ready to hypnotize yourself. But such motives must come from within. You would like to require to modify yourself, not because people think you ought to, but because it's what you would like at the instant.

- **Optimism**

Top people tend not to be skeptics if you're taking a continuum of hypnosis from low to high. This fact does not mean you cannot hypnotize yourself if you're skeptical now. However, we hope that by the top of this subject, your skepticism is going to be alleviated somewhat so that you'll experience hypnosis more easily. It seems that the majority of hypnotic people are likely to possess a hopeful and optimistic view of life. To them, the bottle isn't half empty but half full.

- **Defending**

The people most vulnerable to hypnosis are usually lawyers. This way is often an extension of buoyancy, trust, and hope reflected in their optimism. Whether it's something new in medicine, politics, art, or something that interests them, they're keen to spread the word. Opposite may be a one that is extremely cognitive and scientific in her evaluation. This individual demand evidence wants to read half a dozen books and scrutinizes the topic before committing himself. This attitude of the brain isn't wrong. It simply means such reality-oriented individuals must stay longer in hypnosis to urge results.

- **Concentration**

An important feature of hypnosis is increased concentration. Hypnosis deepens your attention, but you would like it to realize this condition. The more distracting an individual is, the more he responds if he tries to hypnotize himself or is captivated by others. He also has got to use this method more often to form a profit. Meanwhile, most of the people a minimum of sometimes have a deep focus. Attend the space once they are reading and call their name. You cannot get the solution, and those people can't hear your voice because they're too concentrated. We discover no significant evidence difference between vigorous situation and self-hypnosis itself.

- **Acceptability**

Many people are afraid to be hypnotized, not to be absorbed within the will of others. This fact might be called Svengali syndrome. A mysterious stranger with a black cloak and flint's eyes seizes the soul of an unadorned girl while bending her will to adapt to an embarrassing wish. People that are susceptible to hypnosis have normal or good intelligence and a core of beliefs and firm attitudes that are fundamental to life. An example of such an individual is someone with a well-trained religious education that embraces new ideas. He's hard to be fooled. He's sensitive to wise suggestions. Of course, the receptivity level differs from person to person. The receptivity for brand spanking new ideas is one among the determinants of how easily you'll get hypnosis. The main of the population falls within the range 2 to three, on a scale of 0-5 (0 may be a person impervious to hypnosis). However, rest assured that your level of susceptibility to hypnosis isn't included within the five-point scale. At the age of two or three, hypnosis should be repeated more often. However, being at the highest of the size has both disadvantages and benefits.

- **Imagination**

Scientists at the Hypnosis Institute at Stanford University School of Psychology are studying the hypnotic differences between individuals for nearly 20 years. This way is often a project supported by the National psychological state Institute and, therefore, the Air Force Office of Scientific Laboratory. A corporation that doesn't tend to fund little efforts. Dr. Josephine R. Hilgard, a clinical professor of psychiatry at Stanford University, reported on the study: for a few reasons, people that are imaginatively active as a toddler can have hypnosis. The idea states that the imagination and skill to participate in adventures that emerged early in life remained alive and functional through continued use. Among university students, reading, drama, creativity, childhood imagination, religion, sensory, and thirst for adventure were activities identified as hypnosis. Hypnosis is deeply involved in one or more imaginary areas (reading novels, taking note of music, experiencing the aesthetic of nature, adventuring the body and mind) can do. "

Dr. Hilgard found that the scholar in major of humanities is most vulnerable to hypnosis, the majors of social sciences are comparatively less, and students of natural sciences and engineering aren't much hypnotized. The experience and research of other employees during this area tend to corroborate Stanford University results. Consistent with Dr. Lewis R. Wolberg, a 40-year authority within the field: people with the power to enjoy sensory stimulations and may adapt themselves to different roles have more tendency to be hypnotic than others.

Dr. Hilgard's lab was the foremost susceptible to those that had fictitious friends in childhood and will read, adventure, and be immersed in nature. Suspicious, withdrawn, and hostile people have discovered that they tend to resist hypnosis. "Few people appreciate all of the above criteria. You do not even need to show improvement in altogether areas. You'll structure for what's missing in another category. Defined these criteria, hypnosis still needs an excellent deal of research, and it's been accepted by the tutorial and medical profession as a topic that deserves serious investigation. Tons of eye-widening results are drawn from the study.

Why Your Body Gains Weight?

People become emotionally attached to food from infancy through adulthood. Children sometimes get rewarded with snacks or treats for healthy behavior; adults are often treated to dinner. There are numerous celebrations across the year from Christmas, Halloween, Thanksgiving, birthdays, and Valentine Day. of these celebrations are food-focused. As people eat together, they feel good and happy.

It has also been proven that an aroma of a special quite baked cake can create an emotional connection memory which will last throughout someone's lifetime. Some foods are for nourishment, but others we take only for comfort, counting on how they create us feel. Whenever the brain reacts and feels pleasure for a specific food within our reach, most of the time, we'll grab it and eat it. During this point, the brain releases a chemical called dopamine, the method feels perfect, and if we equate the sensation with food, then the result is going to be negative.

High body mass index (BMI) is often linked to emotional problems like anxiety, depression, and stress. Those emotional issues can make one overindulge after a rough day at the office as a gift for an honest feeling. Some people use junks as a coping mechanism once they hear bad news. This habit is often only be improved by the utilization of meditation exercises to affect one's emotions, stress, or anxiety. Because the practices continue, and you pay close attention to your breath and allocate longer for thinking.

Types of Eating

We eat to survive, and without food, we'll die. Our body needs nutrients to function effectively. Eating because one is hungry is different from eating because there's food or one that desires to eat.

We need to coach our system in such how that we eat to curb hunger just a similar way we drink water to quench thirst. While food lovers explore different sorts of food, most of them are keen enough to include healthy eating in their diet.

Mindful Eating

This way is a framework wont to bring back one's relationship with food and eating experiences. During this technique, your presence is significant, and every one the senses are engaged. As an example, how the food smells, the taste of the food, how appetizing it's, and lastly, your body's reaction to the feed.

By this, I mean how that specific food made you are feeling. Mindful eating always incorporates intuitive eating. It makes the body relax and hamper a touch bit as we hear the inner cues of real hunger.

Thus, helping us rectify and reduce emotional binge or emotional eating. Mindful eating can cause weight loss as long together makes the proper food choices. It's a way of eating that's psychologically controlled, and therefore the food portion measured counting on need. In mind eating, it doesn't matter what proportion of food is there.

What matters is that the quantity needed at that specific time. Eating thus becomes a response to hunger aside from a leisure activity. Rarely, People that follow this eating method suffer from obesity. They're physically fit and healthy. During eating also there's no rush, no matter whether one is late or not. The chewing is simultaneous and swallowing.

Intuitive Eating

It is a non-diet approach, mind, and body approach to wellness and health. This approach doesn't encourage dieting but emphasizes taking note of the inner body and hunger cues. By trusting our bodies, intuitive healing renews our relationship with food.

Though it doesn't encourage dieting, it uses nutritional information to form healthy eating choices and habits. By this habit, we eat because we'd like to not because we've to, and dietary values are accepted disinterestedly. During this method, we rely more on our intuition. Food is employed to satisfy a requirement. Without the inner cue of hunger, no need for food. For those that want to flee the strain of dieting can appreciate this approach since it's useful and practical. There's no connection between emotions and food during this sort of eating.

Emotional or Stress Eating

It happens when people start overeating or under food once they are overwhelmed with mixed emotions instead of eating in response to their inner cues. Strong emotions we experience can sometimes prevent us from taking note of our physical feelings and thus preventing us from feeling hungry or full.

In such a scenario, food is employed as a mechanism of coping, thus reducing the effect of extreme emotion temporarily. This habit is extremely addictive, and if not controlled, can cause obesity, rapid weight gain, overeating, guilt, and shame. Stress-related disorder, it cannot handle, can make one vulnerable and not comfortable with the body condition.

This way is where meditation plays a big role because one is going to be ready to handle their stress situation and, therefore, not use food as a coping mechanism.

Stress eating affects many people annually, and although not many will admit it can cause food addiction and unhealthy eating choices. Together eats, they believe diet relieve them of stress and sometimes blame people for his or her problems. They are doing not take responsibility for his or her actions.

They do not see the necessity to eat healthy because their mind is preoccupied with numerous things.

Dieting

Dieting only changes the food you eat for a short time and limit your mindset.

Thus, meditation will assist you in tapping into your inner feelings and answering your craving with the power to regulate yourself.

Not being during a diet also causes you to keep your focus because you'll be keen on what you eat and the way beneficial it's to your body. Meditation for weight loss changes the perception of the mind, which successively triggers the inner self to reply to the alternatives and decisions made. Dieting is restrictive and specific on the meals you're to eat.

It challenges the mind to believe that restriction in terms of food is the only path to weight loss. Meditation, however, may be a healthy way of letting the thought be liberal to choose what's best, learn from mistakes, and be ready to specialize in becoming better. It's possible to realize weight loss once one stops the diet process. It offers both future and short-term weight loss needs. However, the disadvantage is you want to know the calories to require per serving. If you are doing not know, you'll take less, and your body is going to be bereft of the needed nutrient.

The Advantage of a Healthy Body

It is essential to take care of a healthy body to take care of achieves a healthy life. A healthy body enables one to steer a lively and more productive life, which directly translates to great achievements and also age gracefully. To take care of a healthy body, one has got to have a healthy diet, subject himself/herself to regular exercises, maintain a stress-free mind, have a quality sleep and also, lead a healthy lifestyle. The subsequent are ten important reasons for maintaining a healthy body.

- **Boosts the system**

A healthy body means all the body processes are performing at their best, and thus all required antibodies for fighting illness are produced in enough amounts. This way, the body can repel diseases and protect the body from getting sick. Albeit the body cannot resist all illnesses, a healthy body is probably going to repel most seasonal illnesses compared to the non-healthy body. It's advised, however, that if the body's system goes down, it's important to avoid consuming alcohol or taking in food and drinks that are sugary as microbes have a high affinity for sugar.

- **Reduces chances of getting any sort of cancer**

A biological explanation is that the disease of cancer is due to the uncontrolled division of cells, caused to a mutation of the DNA within cells. DNA is liable for giving cells instruction on when to divide, what proportion cells to divide, and also repair cells that require repair. When the DNA mutates, the cells divide uncontrollably and not perform the specified tasks resulting in cancer. Causes of DNA mutations are either inherited genetically, biologically predisposed through chemicals causing disease or unhealthy lifestyles like poor diet, smoking, consumption of loads amounts of alcohol, and obesity. Unhealthy lifestyles are the amount one explanation for cancer. A healthy body contains a traditional DNA, which suggests a controlled cellular division and also, proper repair of cells. it's therefore important to take care of a healthy body

- **Increases the body energy state**

A healthy body has high levels of energy, which are as a result of the work put in to realize it—being healthy means having a healthy diet. A healthy diet means the body is furnished with the specified vitamins, carbohydrates, and proteins required.

Exercising makes the body adapt to harsh treatment, and reciprocally, every exercise session leaves the frame even stronger than it had been before. Enough sleep clears the mind and also gets obviate fatigue. This compilation ultimately translates to the body having high energy levels and more productive.

- **Reduces chances of being infertile**

Being overweight or underweight can increase one chance of being infertile. Also, the abuse of recreational drugs and smoking can contribute greatly to infertility. Being overweight, smoking, and consuming a lot of alcohol in men reduce the sperm count resulting in infertility. Both being underweight and overweight in women also contributes to infertility. All the above-stated problems are a result of an unhealthy body. Therefore, eating healthy to avoid underweight, exercising to curb obesity and overweight cases, and leading a healthy lifestyle and minting a healthy body can go an extended way within the cure for infertility.

- **Prevents stroke and heart-related problems**

Stroke is where the brain is bereft of oxygen for a short time, causing death to its cells. Deprivation of oxygen could also be caused by blockage of arteries or rupturing of arteries resulting in leakage of oxygenated blood liable for keeping cells up and running. Among the causes of blocked arteries is thanks to the deposition of fat blocking the right flow of blood to the brain. Other causes may include unhealthy lifestyles and stress. Heart problems include attack and arteria coronaria disease.

Similarly, arteria coronaria disease is caused by an excessive amount of cholesterol, blocking the availability of blood to the body. An attack is that the rapture of the coronary artery; it's as a result of the guts pumping blood at a better rhythmic pressure than the traditional one. This way creates pressure on the artery, causing them to rapture. The simplest treatment approved by doctors for both diseases is exercising, leading a healthy lifestyle, having enough rest, avoiding stress, and also adopting a healthy diet. Doctors stress keeping our bodies healthy as we are ready to repel illnesses like heart problems and stroke, among others.

- **Enhances some career choices**

Careers like athletics require athletes to take care of healthy living standards and impressive body physique. Athletes are required to adopt a strict diet, exercise regularly, and subject their bodies to enough sleep and, most of all, avoid consumption of recreational drugs also as an excessive amount of alcohol if not a little amount. Within the show business, too, models and dancers are mostly required to stick to similar living standards. These healthy standards ensure their bodies are at optimum health, and that they are ready to remain top of their careers.

- **Improves longevity**

Study within time has shown that having a healthy body ensures one realizes a long life. Exercising as little as twenty minutes each day reduced the probabilities of 1 suffering a premature death. Healthy adjustments like proper diet also are essential in achieving an extended life. The healthy body, even at an older age, also means one is in a position to hold out tasks that might are hard if they were unhealthy or dead. It also means one is in a place to enjoy longer with family. Grandparents get an opportunity to ascertain and bond with their grandchildren all due to maintaining their bodies at healthy levels

- **Helps control weight**

A healthy body may be a state acquired after proper care of the body and exercises. Even without trying to reduce, robust living standards will ultimately cause a healthy weight. A weekly schedule of a couple of hours of training and eating right will go an extended way in maintaining a healthy weight. The body will have a robust system, prevent heart diseases and also spike the body energy state all as a result of a healthy body

- **Improves moods and feelings**

A study has proven that exercising our body leaves our bodies relaxed and happy also. This way is often a result of the discharge of nerve cell chemicals called endorphins. Training also ensures that one achieves an athletic physique, which suggests that one will have improved physical appearances resulting in enhanced self-confidence. We sleep in a world of constant disappointments and tragedies. it's essential to stay out bodies at the most health for improved emotional balance and also maximum cognitive functions

- **Helps manage diabetes**

There are two primary sorts of diabetes, type one where the body insulin-producing cells are attacked itself, by the body. Then you'll need to survive insulin shots all his/ her life. Type two diabetes is where the body is unable to soak up the sugar within the blood and convert it into energy for the cells. Type one diabetes may be a result of poor health living standards, lack of exercise, and having poor diet. A correct diet and exercise often control the early stages of diabetes like Pre diabetes and also gestational diabetes. Maintaining a healthy body will mean that the body is going to be ready to control body insulin balance and reduce fatalities caused by diabetes like a vital sign, attack, renal failure, and hardening of blood vessels

- **Improves the brains memory**

A healthy body constitutes a healthy diet; a healthy diet comprises of all the food nutrients. Among these nutrients are vitamins. Vitamins, preferably C, E, D, Omega 3, fatty acids, and flavonoids, are essential in developing a brain with an honest memory. A healthy diet also helps repel dementia and decline of cognitive functions. Dementia is that the loss of consciousness, effects on the power to talk, think, or maybe solve a drag. Eating healthy will help reduce dementia that which isn't caused by physical injury on the brain.

- **Strengthens the bones and the teeth.**

Maintaining a healthy body helps improve the strength of teeth and bones. It's advisable to consume dairy products for calcium three portions each day. One is additionally required to subject the body to physical exercises, and therefore the most preferred one is lifting weights. A correct diet is essential, as well. One is required to consume meals rich in calcium and magnesium for stronger teeth and bones. Many sorts of cereal contain calcium while magnesium is abundantly found in legumes, nuts, whole grains and seeds

- **Boosts self-esteem**

Among reasons for having low self-esteem has an unhealthy body. We sleep in a world of diversity and one that's rich in several tastes in fashion. Often everyone wants to seem right, but sometimes our bodies often fail us, and this will be bad for our self-esteem. However, this will be changed, and our esteem boosted within no time. A correct diet would be an honest start amid regular body exercises and maintaining a healthy mind through rest and controlling what we expect. Results take time, but eventually, one achieves a healthy body. This way is often more like killing two birds with one stone together is in a position to spice up their self-confidence by enhancing appearances and also achieve a state of a healthy body through having a healthy body.

- **A Healthy body improves better sleep**

Often people with unhealthy bodies undergo tons of difficulties when sleeping. They often sweat tons in cases of obesity and even find problems breathing when asleep. Healthy people sleep well and encounter no problems breathing when sleeping. Subjecting the body to exercises ensures the bodily process work right, and it burns off excess fats causing sweating during the night. Eating right and avoiding abuse of medicine and alcohol also helps achieve a healthy body. A healthy body, in turn, results in sound sleep

- **Improves sex life in couples**

Sex may be a physical act; it's therefore required for both partners to be physically slotted to possess a reasonable time. More often than not, once one among the partners gains an unreasonable amount of weight or both of the partners, they begin experiencing bedroom problems. Sex may be a significant aspect of all couples, and if issues arise during this area, the likelihood of separation is high. It's therefore advised of couples that they maintain healthy bodies to avoid bedroom problems.

- **Improves chances of surviving disasters and violence**

We sleep in the 21st century, where the planet may be a subject of natural disasters also as man inflicted violence's from robbery to wars. The earth is not any longer a secure place, and nobody is an exemption to the present bitter truth. So, just in case of an onset of such misfortunes, the citizenry is alleged to find ways to survive. Among methods of improving the probabilities of survival in such cases has a healthy body, both strong and athletic. The rule of life would take the course, and therefore the strong and fit that healthy people are getting to survive. A healthy person is more likely to evade himself/herself from a scene of violence by moving away as quickly as possible. An unhealthy person won't be so lucky.

Tackling Barriers to Weight Loss

There are numerous barriers to weight loss from personal, to medical, to network and emotional health. Meditation, if incorporated, will bring fruitful and healthy results. Dedication to beat the challenges and to be focused on achieving your goals is critical. There are numerous distractions, especially before you begin tour weight loss routine.

It takes discipline and resilience to manage a healthy loss program. We'd like to offer weight loss the priority it deserves. Also, we'd like to understand the existence of the said barriers and their contribution toward our goal. The walls will determine our successes and failures.

Set realistic goals

When you set goals, make sure that they're attainable, specific, and realistic. It's effortless to figure on realistic goals and achieve them for better results. If the goals are unrealistic, the success rate is going to be low and is going to be discouraged. As an example, when starting with meditation, you'll start with as little as five minutes each day and gradually increase it daily until you reach the whole time like sixty minutes.

The same applies to reduce during the meditation process. You'll start that specialize in losing a couple of pounds hebdomadally and gradually increase until you reach your goal. As you set goals, however, realize that it's not your fault if they are doing not compute as you had planned, do your best and keep your focus.

Always be accountable

Once you've got decided to plan to meditation to weight loss, don't recoil from sharing your plan with your network and family. It's to make sure that the people you share with also reinforce the commitment and form a part of the system. That way, they're going to feel a part of the program and provides support whenever there's a requirement. You'll also use apps for reminders and timings; this manner, you've got a backup plan whenever you forget.

You can also use motivational bands whenever you achieve a milestone set. Being accountable causes you to enjoy your successes, acknowledge your failure, and appreciate your network.

People thrive once they feel liable for something, especially on something beneficial to their well-being.

Modify your mindset

Your thinking must be modified within the sense that you simply be keen on the knowledge you're telling yourself. Make sure that your mind isn't crammed with unproductive and negative thoughts, which can bring you down or discourage you. Don't be frightened of challenging your ideas and appreciate your body image.

Your mindset determines your thinking and successively, creates a way of appreciation or rejection. Our weight loss largely depends on our mindset, does one believe you'll do it? If you think that you've got all it takes, then absolutely nothing will prevent or stop you.

Manage stress regularly

Having a stress management technique should be a part of one's daily routine. You would like to develop a healthy stress-relieving mechanism that will assist you in living a stress-free life. Understand that meditation may be a stress reliever in its title because it helps calm the mind and soothes the body.

It is often wont to manage stress and its benefits fully utilized to measure a more productive life. Be ready to handle stress efficiently. The pressure isn't healthy for the mind.

If not handle, it can cause emotional problems and makes one irrational, moody, or violent. Be your boss when managing your stress.

Be educated about weight loss

Suppose you start meditation for weight loss then be educated about how it works; that way, weight loss won't be a struggle.

You will be ready to handle failed attempts also appreciate the progress made.

You will be ready to know what you've got been doing wrong and choose the simplest meditation exercise for you.

If you've got misleading information, then your general progress could also be inhibited

Weight loss needn't be too expensive; neither does it require a costly gym membership or enrolment during a costly meditation class. There are various self-practice meditation exercises that you can comfortably do the reception . There are multiple meal plans and diets which will work for others though they'll not offer future solutions or lasting behavior changes. Have the proper information that you simply need. Do not be misled by anyone posing that they're professionals therein field. Also, don't hesitate to try to research online and compare notes. From there, you'll be ready to come with something that works for you.

Surround yourself with a network

There are people out there who could also be ready and willing to assist whenever you would like to start out or maybe after you've got started.

The network may include your family, colleagues, friends, or social networks. These groups of wonderful people may encourage and support you to satisfy your long-term goal. After you include them in your plan, they're going to feel accepted, offer opinions, and check on your progress. Analyze how things are going, also as encourage you to continue taking a touch break when necessary.

Your network should also include professionals within the field who will give sound advice and offer needed support and care.

They will also assist you in discovering the items hindering you and holding you behind also as offer reliable information that will help you overcome. As you decide on the professional you would like to figure with, ensure they're people that are easy to speak to. People that are willing to be a participant within the routine you select. You'll also consider people that can give an honest opinion also as recommendations. Support systems sometimes have similar challenges that you simply could even be browsing at that specific time.

Their words of encouragement and best wishes usually would go an extended way in motivating someone. Realize that ideologies may correspond together with your point of view.

Overcoming Mental Blocks to Lose Weight

What beliefs are holding onto your weight?

I am inferior

I am lacking

I am inconsequential, so I even have to form myself big to be seen

Losing weight is just too difficult

I will fail and put the load all back on again

I must be so awful and bad not to be ready to control my eating

I want to punish myself

It is too hard to start dieting

My weight is ancestral, and that I can't change that

My weight is genetic, and that I can't change that

I am not good enough/I am not enough

I self-sabotage myself

I am worthless

I loathe myself

Healing Negative Beliefs

The best ways to improve negative beliefs and build confidence are:

- Emotional Freedom Technique (EFTTM) –
- Bach Flower Remedies
- Affirmations
- Ask your guides and angels to assist and heal you

A pattern may be a program that you simply have, which is a component of your personality. for instance, in your character might be the thoughts:

I am not nearly as good as people

This fact means that you block your weight loss as you feel that the task is just too daunting, and you'll fail. New patterns are often easily installed using EFTTM.

A block is some things that stop you moving forward, and therefore the biggest one among these is FEAR. The opposite one is safe. If your subconscious feels that it's not safe, it'll NOT allow you to roll in the hay. So, if your subconscious thinks that losing weight isn't safe, you'll NOT LOSE WEIGHT!

Also, if you think that you're worthless, otherwise you feel you are doing not deserve, this may cause you to self-sabotage.

Healing Negative Patterns and Blocks

The best ways to treat negative patterns and blocks are:

- Emotional Freedom Technique

- Bach Flower Remedies
- Affirmations
- Meditation
- Ask your guides and angels to assist and heal you
- What is self-sabotage?

The term self-sabotage describes our often-unconscious ability to prevent ourselves from being, doing, or having, being the person we would like to be, doing what we would like to experience or achieve, or having our goals and desires become a reality.

Most of the time, we are totally unaware that we are self-sabotaging because it happens on a subconscious level. However, sometimes we are conscious of that tiny voice within the back of our head that says, "you can't learn a language" or "don't be ridiculous, you can't lose weight."

Our subconscious may be a powerful tool and always thinks that it's acting in our greatest interest. Stopping us getting into new territory, discouraging us from taking risks ensures that we don't get hurt, we aren't humiliated, and that we don't fail – that's why numerous projects never get off the bottom. Instead of playing to win, self-sabotage plays to avoid defeat.

The purpose of this aspect of the subconscious is self-protection and survival. It can even negatively affect your health if it thinks that this may protect you from greater risk. Layers of excess weight have long been recognized as protection. Really often the subconscious will use weight gain to guard you against perceived dangers you would possibly be exposed to as a slimmer person. for instance, where someone has been abused as a toddler, the subconscious may add weight to form them unattractive (it thinks) so that the abuse isn't repeated.

So, people may mention self-sabotage about their weight because they ate emotionally and placed on weight. However, sometimes self-sabotage will affect your hormones and/or organs, causing weight gain in people that eat only a modest amount. Sometimes people can reduce but always put it back on just another method of self-sabotage. Once the perceived got to protect through self-sabotage has been healed and released, our illnesses and weight may disappear.

My Experience of Self-Sabotage

In my quest to lose the load and water I had accumulated, I consulted a woman who specialized in 'muscle testing.' Once we asked the question "Do I would like to be slim," the apparent reply was "no!" which took me all of a sudden. So then started the journey of discovery on why my subconscious didn't want me to be slim.

Why was I self-sabotaging?

During the long seventeen years during which I slowly cleared and healed the explanations for my self- sabotage:

I had found out a self-punishment/self-destruct program due to what I had wiped out past lives

I had found out protection around me (weight and water) due to the sexual assault, rape and male attention I had had – I didn't feel it had been safe to be a lady

I had several past life issues with starving to death and didn't want to starve during this lifetime

I had several past life issues with dying of thirst, hence the surplus water during this lifetime to make sure that it didn't happen again

I had an incredible amount of other karma

I thought that if I became a therapist, I couldn't trust myself not to hurt, or experiment on patients, as I had cut them before in past lives, then I used to be only getting to be a therapist once I was 'slim.'

I was frightened to require herbs as I had seen numerous people die from them in past lives

Because I had been persecuted in past lives for healing people, I assumed that I might be abused during this life; also, I used to be scared of being powerful

I was frightened to try to work I used to be alleged to do

I was frightened that the book would fail

I relate to my self-sabotage with weight and health, but there have been many other areas of my life that affected.

I was always in debt and will never pay off my credit cards

I never got the work I deserved and was reasonably often out of the labor

If I got employment, there would always be someone giving me a troublesome time (karmic payback!)

When I had any treatments, like red vein treatment or cosmetic surgery, it might always fail

Believe it or not, my subconscious was creating a reality where all of the above occurred – the psyche is that strong, believe me. Even once I had released the attachments and got obviate the influence of my mother, my subconscious was still following their examples, and as I strived to urge better, my subconscious kicked in and made it worse.

So, my subconscious was actually affecting all my organs and making them inefficiently work so that I placed on six stone and swelled up with water. This fact was because my subconscious knew I could reduce, and it decided this was the simplest plan of attack.

That's why some people reduce then put it back on. The subconscious doesn't always realize what's happening to start with, hence the load loss. It then kicks in success in survival mode, and therefore the weight goes back on. You'd not lose six stone then put it back on again – you would possibly replace a stone then catch on-off. People blame diets or losing it too quickly, but it's merely your subconscious sabotaging you.

Emotional and Luxury Eating

When you read magazine articles, they always mention emotional eating and weight gain. Some people do eat for psychological reasons and tedium. Some people do overeat, and there are explanations for this. You would like to spot your emotional eating triggers and use of a way like EFTtm to eliminate them. However, if you would like to eat an attempt to wait 10 minutes breathing deeply and you ought to find that, then the necessity to eat has gone.

However, I do know tons of slim people that overeat and drink an excessive amount of. They eat more for emotional reasons also – thin people aren't perfect or without their problems.

One of the explanations I wrote this book is to point out that overweight people don't eat emotionally any longer than slim/ordinary people. How often are you on holiday and you watch people eat a huge breakfast, followed by a huge lunch then three courses for dinner, plus booze, a day for two weeks? How often does one see a slim person eat a packet of biscuits or a bar of chocolate? ALL THE TIME!

You have to seek out the explanations why your subconscious doesn't want to reduce and either release the descriptions if these are past lives based or change your subconscious 'belief system' if they're more personality traits.

Removing the Self-Sabotage

When I was spending an enormous amount of cash with therapists and zip worked, I did mention that I'd be self-sabotaging myself. Most of them threw their hands up in horror and told me it had been just an excuse to overeat (here we return, I thought).

I read tons about the Emotional Freedom Technique (EFTTM), and within the very first paragraph, I read it mentioned self-sabotage. This way was quite fantastic. However, my self-sabotage was so deeply ingrained that for an extended time,

EFTTM just made everything worse, as my subconscious tried to carry onto its control of me.

I, therefore, had to dig much deeper by clearing the attachments, past lives, and karma, then I could use EFTTM and my other techniques to vary my subconscious perception and its belief system that "I didn't deserve."

Psychological reversal

I thought that I wanted to reduce, but I didn't, and my subconscious was stopping me. You would like to seek out all the explanations of why and release and heal them one by one. For this, you employ the EFTTM psychological reversal techniques.

How are you self-sabotaging because my experience would lead me to believe that you simply are?

Habit of self-sabotage

I had a spiritual reading session and was told that the self-punishment had been healed but that I still had the 'habit' which needed to be treated and not recreated. I feel it's vital to incorporate it during this book because it would haven't occurred to me that I still had the habit and was capable of recreating the practice at any time. Our body and subconscious sabotage us such a lot that it becomes automatic than a practice. So even when the first stimuli are healed, the habit remains. So, remember to check to ascertain whether there's a habit then treat accordingly (normally a similar way you healed the first pattern). Confirm you don't recreate the practice by repeating affirmations and if you are feeling yourself slipping back to 'deserving the pattern' immediately cancel this sense and make sure that you retain healing it.

What is the secondary gain?

Believe it or not, every illness and problem can have a significant benefit for the one that is experiencing it. Professionals use the term 'secondary gain' for this well-known phenomenon, and you'll start to acknowledge this behavior in folks that you recognize. In some cases, the advantages of getting the matter are so great they outweigh the suffering the thing is causing.

This problem is made by the subconscious, totally unbeknown to the person. Often this person pushing themselves too hard, and therefore the unconscious will come up with how to affect what's happening there in person's life, so an illness or a drag is made that's not under their control.

A good question to ask yourself is, "what are the advantages to you that this illness or the matter brings, and why are you keeping it around?". So, what are the advantages of you holding onto the surplus weight? Analyze this question very carefully and dig until you get to the rock bottom of it.

Some samples of secondary gain:

- You have hurt your leg, but it stops you from doing something you don't like, and you get many sympathies – a double whammy!
- You placed on weight, and this stops you going out of the house and your entire family are worried about you and fuss over you

- A friend takes care of a relative and is usually rushing around after them. All her friends tell her how marvelous and dedicated she is, so she, in turn, gets many attention and sympathy that wouldn't get if she stopped does one recognize yourself here?

Watch your thoughts!

Watch your thoughts, for they become your words.

Watch your words, for they become your actions.

Watch your actions for they become your habits.

Watch your habits, for they become your character.

Watch your character, for it becomes your destiny.

Your subconscious believes everything it hears!

Remember that your subconscious listens to what's said to you by people or yourself, and it takes everything it hears literally. It cannot differentiate between a joke and reality, so never put yourself down, during a fun. So, if you retain telling yourself that you are FAT, your subconscious will cause you to fat and keep you that way. Your fat cells will think – I'm fat, so I better keep my cells nicely plumped up and not lose them. Yes, this is often really true!

I know it sounds amusing, but often this is what happens in the real world, and therefore the beautiful poem displayed at the highest of the page becomes your reality – and what you think becomes your truth.

We mention beliefs tons during this book and changing them from being negative to positive – so we are watching positive thinking here—the half-full glass instead of the half-empty glass.

I was told I used to be fat, stupid, and ugly from the first moment I remember, and thus that's what I believed. Even once I lost weight, I still thought I used to be fat, and since I projected that outwards people treated as if I were still fat too. Now once I check out pictures of myself as a plump child or a slim adult, I feel that really I'm beautiful, perhaps a touch large but never fat, stupid, or ugly.

Once I was on holiday there was a touch Italian girl on the beach – she was quite understandable. All the adults around her kept calling her beautiful and smart and had such a smile that showed that she believed it.

This belief would follow her into adulthood, and she or he would believe that she was beautiful, slim, and smart for the remainder of her life and that I think this is often absolutely brilliant! I assumed how wonderful of those people to instill such fabulous qualities in one so young. In our day, we were never ok, never lived up to expectations – were a disappointment. Never were we told that our parents loved us and that I still know people to the present day who try to urge their parent's approval – albeit they're over fifty.

I will never say anything negative to anyone, including someone young – they're always beautiful, great and smart and that I am still pleased with them – I wish someone had told me that they were delighted with me.

Talking About Yourself

So, you want to mention yourself with positive beliefs, albeit you don't believe them at the time – fake it until you create it (as is that the current phrase!) and within the case of weight problems, think sort of a slim person. A lover of mine who had placed on tons of weight said that she was surprised when she saw an image of herself at that point, as believed she was still slim – so it does work both ways!

Most people who usually are overweight are very critical and always speak negatively about themselves. They typically suffer from low self-worth and low self-esteem. The result's that, by doing this, they're perpetuating the matter. Once you are speaking negatively to yourself, ask yourself if you'd talk to a love like that. The solution most likely is going to be that you directly wouldn't, so why on earth are you speaking like that to yourself? Stop it now!

It is almost impossible for your body to vary once you keep sending it negative messages. As long as you say, "I am FAT," you give your body more instruction and energy to BE FAT.

It would help if you varied your chatter from negative to positive, albeit you don't believe what you're saying. I hear you cry, "How am I able to be positive once I am fat?" but it's vital within the re-programming of your subconscious and your cells. Positive affirmations are a superb way of re-programming, and these are often combined with EFTTM for stronger and quicker results.

Change 'I am fat' to 'I get slimmer every day.'

Change 'I never lose weight' to 'It gets easier a day to lose weight.'

Changing Beliefs

People ask how they will change their beliefs, and fortunately, lately, there's a spread of techniques and therapies to assist and do that, but you furthermore may need to take care not to fall back to any bad habits.

This way relates to all or any areas in your life and not just to weight, so let me tell you a few stories:

I love Sunday nights as this is often my pamper night, where I even have an extended bath, mask, and do my nails. A number of my friends hate Sunday night because they need to travel back to the figure on Monday and that they don't like their jobs. I even have changed my perception of Sunday night so that I enjoy it, unlike my friends who dread it.

Forgiving Yourself for Your Dietary Mistakes

Forgiveness is an underrated and essential element of weight loss. Often, people that are within the position of wanting or wanting to reduce and fail to acknowledge the very fact that they need been feeling incredibly frustrated with themselves. Anger, frustration, disappointment, and sadness directed at yourself once you are on this journey are all incredibly normal feelings to possess.

They can even be painful and overwhelming if you are doing not take the time to acknowledge them, forgive yourself, and heal them as you experience them.

You may end up feeling angry, frustrated, disappointed, or sad that you simply let yourself gain such a lot of weight. You'll fail to acknowledge the very fact that it had been not intentional, or that it had causes that were beyond your control, mainly if your weight gain was associated with medical conditions or a scarcity of education around healthy eating.

Regardless of what causes you to gain weight, you'll feel contempt for yourself for “allowing” it to happen, which may make it difficult for you to plan to lose weight.

When you sit in anger and frustration with yourself, it is often difficult to simply accept yourself as you're now and work toward improving your wellbeing through weight loss. Forgiving yourself for not knowing better or for not doing better, or maybe forgiving yourself for blaming yourself for something that was beyond your control, is vital.

The more you'll forgive yourself, the more likely you're to acknowledge that your weight is some things you would like to figure on. Through that, you'll be ready to work on weight loss from a peaceful frame of mind.

Studies have shown that those that accept themselves as they're and forgive their mistakes are more likely to lose the surplus weight and keep it off than those that refuse to forgive themselves. Refusing to forgive yourself can create a huge amount of stress inside you that creates it difficult for you to remain focused on exercising, eating healthy, and improving your wellness. Many of us find that this difficulty in forgiving themselves worsens their self-esteem and self-confidence, which keeps them within the unhealthy cycle of behaviors and patterns that cause their weight gain within the first place. If you would like to beat these cycles, you would like to be willing to forgive yourself for your past choices, mistakes, and experiences which will or might not are beyond your control.

Another area where you would like to master forgiveness is within the process of change. As you progress faraway from old habits and behaviors and into a replacement way of taking care of your body, you're about bound to make mistakes.

You are getting to have days or maybe weeks where you fall back to old patterns.

Some people even fall back to old patterns and stay trapped in them for years. This fact happens because they're unwilling to forgive themselves for creating an error, then they fall back to the cycle of contempt and low self-esteem and self-worth.

If you would like to be ready to continue moving forward together with your wellness and to leap back on target as quickly as possible, you would like to be willing to forgive yourself for any mistakes you create.

This way means anytime you overeat, engage in an old eating pattern, choose an unhealthy food choice, or otherwise make a “mistake” in your diet, and you forgive yourself. Upon forgiving yourself, confirm that you also plan to take that have under consideration so that you'll make better choices. Make an honest effort to try to do better next time so that whenever you forgive yourself, you give yourself a reason to believe that your commitment to yourself genuinely means something.

When you can forgive yourself and believe that your commitment to bettering yourself and your life means something, you start to create your self-esteem. Through that, things like portion control begin to become easier, and you discover yourself naturally gravitating toward taking better care of yourself.

Meditation for Portion Control

The following may be a simple 5-10-minute meditation that you simply can do before you sit right down to eat a meal.

Using it's getting to assist you intentionally engage in portion control in order that you'll refrain from overeating.

Adding this meditation into the mixture will make sure that you're approaching your improved portion control from a deep subconscious level, allowing you to experience even more success in committing to moderation and healing your body through weight loss.

When you do that meditation, you ought to be actively sitting up with a straight spine. Laying down may cause you feeling too tired or creating excess calmness in your day, which can cause you to struggle to take care of energy throughout the day.

The Meditation

I want you to start by intentionally taking one sweet deep breath into your belly, pressing your belly button and chest forward together with your breath. Then, once you exhale, let your belly button and chest drawback toward your spine. Feel the movement of your body because it naturally flows with each breath.

Do not attempt to control the speed at which you breathe, but instead feel how your body naturally breathes in and out for you. Feel your body intuitively drawing in and circulating oxygen throughout your body, and exhaling CO2 from your body even as easily.

Notice how calm your body feels with each breath. Feel how breathing is so natural, so simple, so basic, and yet continues to be one among the strongest stress relievers we've. Meditate here together with your breath for a couple of moments as you sink deeply into this sense of trusting your body. In this way your intuition to require care of you thru each breath.

Now, I would like you to draw your awareness even deeper, into your stomach. Pause for a flash and see any hunger which will be arising within your body.

Take into consideration what this hunger seems like and what cues your body is supplying you with that indicates that it's time to eat. Feel yourself acknowledging and becoming conscious of your own needs and trust that your intuition is providing you with the proper information about your body.

As you begin taking note of your intuition about your hunger, ask yourself: "How hungry am I?" concentrate on the solution that rises. Are you hungry for a snack or a full meal? Be mindful of what proportion food your body genuinely wants and the way much it needs.

Now, ask yourself, "what am I actually hungry for?" and pay close attention. Trust that whatever answer comes in is correct and be willing to figure alongside your body to seek out the simplest source of nutrition for you and your wellbeing.

Trust that when you're done this meditation, you'll choose something healthier and more nutritious, which will help your body meet its needs.

As you still sit together with your intuition, develop a trust in your inner knowingness and your emotional ability to acknowledge your hunger cues. Ask your body to be honest about once you feel full and ask it to assist you naturally stop craving food so that you'll stop eating when your body feels full.

Affirm that you simply want to require care of your body and earn its trust by serving it within the way that it truly must be served.

Affirm that you deserve genuinely enjoying healthy portions of food that nourish your body without overwhelming you. Feel yourself being fulfilled and satisfied by these affirmations.

Trust that they're right, which your subconscious, unconscious, and conscious mind can all work together to assist you in managing your eating habits more effectively.

When you are able to awaken yourself from this meditation, bring your awareness back to your breath, then to your body. Feel yourself gently awakening from this moment of peace and permit yourself to acknowledge what your body told you it needed.

Act thereon information and, to the simplest of your ability, follow your intuition and hunger cues to make sure that you simply feed yourself an appropriate amount of healthy, nutritious food.

If, during the meditation, your body informed you that it had been not hungry but instead required emotional support, make sure to avoid emotional eating and instead hunt down an alternate way for managing your emotions. The more you'll practice following these intuitive cues around feelings and other needs, additionally to your hunger cues, the higher you're getting to be ready to look out of yourself.

Through this, you'll end up naturally engaging in portion control and taking care of your wellbeing through your diet. As a result, you'll reduce faster, easier, and in a healthier manner.

Affirmation to Cut Calories

Affirmations are an excellent tool to use alongside hypnosis to assist you in rewiring your brain and improving your weight loss abilities. Statements are essentially a tool that you use to remind you of your chosen "rewiring" and to encourage your mind to select your newer, healthier mindset over your old unhealthy one. Using affirmations is a crucial part of anchoring your hypnosis efforts into your lifestyle, so it's vital that you use them on a routine basis.

When using affirmations, it's important that you simply use relevant ones, which are getting to support you in anchoring your chosen reality into your present reality.

What Are Affirmations, and the Way Do They Work?

Anytime you repeat something to yourself aloud, or in your thoughts, you're affirming something to yourself. We use affirmations consistently, whether we consciously know it or not. For instance, if you're on your weight loss journey and you repeat "I am never getting to lose the weight" to yourself daily, you're affirming to yourself that you only are never getting to succeed with weight loss. Likewise, if you're consistently saying, "I will always be fat" or "I am never getting to reach my goals," you're affirming those things to yourself, too.

When we use affirmations unintentionally, we frequently find ourselves using statements that will be hurtful and harmful to our psyche and our reality.

You might end up locking into becoming a mental bully toward yourself as you consistently repeat things to yourself that are unkind and even downright mean. As you are doing this, you affirm a lower sense of self-confidence, a scarcity of motivation, and a commitment to a body shape and wellness journey that you simply don't want to take care of.

Affirmations, whether positive or negative, conscious, or unconscious, are always creating or reinforcing the function of your brain and mindset.

Each time you repeat something to yourself, your subconscious hears it and strives to form it a neighborhood of your reality. This fact is often because your subconscious is liable for creating your truth and your sense of identity.

It creates both around your affirmations since these are what you perceive as being your absolute truth; therefore, they create a "concrete" foundation for your reality and identity to rest on.

If you would like to vary these two aspects of yourself and your experience, you're getting to got to change what you're routinely repeating to yourself so that you're not creating a reality and identity rooted in negativity.

To vary your subconscious experience, you would like to consciously choose positive affirmations and repeat them continuingly to assist you in achieving the truth and identity that you only genuinely want.

This way, you're more likely to make an experience that reflects what you're trying to find, instead of an experience that reflects what your conscious and subconscious has automatically picked abreast of.

The key with affirmations is that you simply got to understand that your brain doesn't care if you're creating them intentionally or not.

It also doesn't care if you're creating healthy and positive ones or unhealthy and negative ones.

All your subconscious cares about is what's repeated thereto, and what you perceive as being your absolute truth.

It is up to you and your conscious mind to acknowledge that negative and unhealthy affirmations will hold you back, prevent you from experiencing positive experiences in life, and end in you feeling incapable and unmotivated.

Alternatively, consciously choosing healthy and positive affirmations will assist you with creating a healthier mindset and an identity that serves your wellbeing on a mental, physical, emotional, and spiritual level. From there, your responsibility is to repeat these affirmations to yourself until you think them consistently, and you start to ascertain them being reflected in your reality.

How Do I Pick and Use Affirmations for Weight Loss?

Choosing affirmations for your weight loss journey requires you first to understand what it's that you merely are trying to find, and what sorts of positive thoughts are getting to assist you in getting there. You'll start by identifying what your dream is, what you would like your ideal body to seem and desire, and the way you would like to feel as you achieve your thought of losing weight. Once you've got identified what your idea is, you would like to spot what current beliefs you've got round the hope that you simply are meaning to achieve.

For example, if you would like to lose 25 pounds so that you'll have a healthier weight, but you think that it'll be incredibly hard to lose that weight, then you recognize that your current beliefs are that losing weight is tough. You would like to spot every single opinion surrounding your weight loss goals and understand which of them are negative or are limiting and preventing you from achieving your goal of losing weight.

After you've got identified which of your beliefs are negative and unhelpful, you'll choose affirmations that are getting to assist you to change your beliefs. Typically, you would like to settle on a statement that's getting to help you completely change that belief within the other way.

For example, if you think that "losing weight is tough," then your new affirmation might be "I lose the load effortlessly." Albeit you are doing not believe this further affirmation immediately, the goal is to repeat it to yourself enough that it becomes a neighborhood of your identity and, inevitably, your reality. This way, you're anchoring in your hypnosis sessions, and you're effectively rewiring your brain in between sessions, too.

As you employ affirmations to assist you achieve weight loss, I encourage you to try to so during a way that's intuitive to your experience.

There are no right or wrong thanks to approaching affirmations, as long as you're using them daily. Once you are feeling yourself effortlessly believing in a statement, you'll start incorporating new affirmations into your routine so that you'll still use your affirmations to enhance your wellbeing overall. Ideally, you ought to always be using positive affirmations even after you've got seen the changes you desire, as statements are an exquisite thanks to naturally helping maintain your mental, emotional, and physical wellbeing.

What Should I Do with My Affirmations?

After you've got chosen what affirmations you would like to use and which of them are getting to feel best for you, you would like to understand what to try to with them! The only thanks to using your affirmations are to select 1-2 statements and repeat them to yourself daily. You'll repeat them anytime you are feeling the necessity to re-affirm something to yourself;

otherwise, you can repeat them continually, albeit they are doing not seem entirely relevant within the moment.

The keys to making sure that you simply are always repeating them to yourself so that you're more likely to possess success in rewiring your brain and achieving the new, healthier, and simpler beliefs that you got to improve the standard of your life.

In addition to repeating your affirmations to yourself, you'll also use them in many other ways. A method that folks like using statements are by writing them down.

You can write your affirmations down on little notes and leave them around your house; otherwise, you can make a ritual out of writing your statements down a particular amount of times per day during a journal so that you're ready to work them into your day routinely. Some people also will meditate on their affirmations, meaning that they essentially meditate then repeat the affirmations to themselves over and over during a meditative state.

If repeating your affirmation to yourself sort of a mantra is just too challenging, you'll also say your chosen affirmations to yourself on a voice recording track then repeat them to yourself on loop while you meditate.

Other people will create recordings of themselves repeating several affirmations into their voice recorder then taking note of them on loop. At the same time, they compute, eat, drive to figure, or otherwise engage in an activity where affirmations could be useful.

If you want to form your affirmations productive and obtain the foremost out of them, you would like to seek out how to bombard your brain with this new information necessarily. The more effectively you'll do that, the more your subconscious mind goes to select abreast of it and still reinforce your new neural pathways with these new affirmations. Through that, you'll end up effortlessly and naturally believing within the new statements that you simply have chosen for yourself.

How Are Affirmations Going to Help Me Lose Weight?

Affirmations are getting to assist you in reducing during a few alternative ways. First and foremost, and doubtless most blatant, is that the indisputable fact that statements are arriving to help you get within the mindset of weight loss.

To put it simply: you can't sit around believing nothing goes to figure and expect things to think for you. You would like to be ready to cultivate a motivated mindset that permits you to make success. If you're unable to believe that it'll come true: trust that it'll not come true.

As your mindset improves, your subconscious is getting to start changing other things within your body, too.

For example, instead of creating desires and cravings for things that aren't healthy for you, your body will begin to make desires and cravings for items that are healthy for you. It'll also stop creating inner conflict around making the proper choices and taking care of yourself. You'll even end up falling crazy together with your new diet and your new exercise routine.

You will also likely end up naturally leaning toward behaviors and habits that are healthier for you without having to undertake so hard to make those habits. In many cases, you would possibly create practices that are healthy for you without even realizing that you simply are creating those habits.

Rather than having to consciously become conscious of the necessity for habits, then fixing the work to make them, your body and mind will naturally begin to acknowledge the need for better practices and can create those habits usually also.

Some studies have also suggested that using affirmations will help your brain and subconscious govern your body differently, too. For instance, you'll be ready to improve your body's ability to digest things and manage your weight naturally by using affirmations and hypnosis. In doing so, you'll be prepared to subconsciously adjust which hormones, chemicals, and enzymes are created within your body to assist with things like digestive functions, energy creation, and other weight- and health-related concerns that you may have.

You can use these affirmations as there; otherwise, you can adjust them to match what you would like for your belief system. If you are doing rewrite them, confirm that you simply are creating ones that directly reflect what you would like to listen to so that you'll change your beliefs to ones that are more supportive and fewer limiting.

Affirmations for Self-Control

Self-control is a crucial discipline to possess, and not having it can cause behaviors that are known for creating weight loss tougher. If you're battling self-control, the subsequent affirmations will assist you in changing any beliefs you've got around restraint so that you'll start approaching food, exercise, weight loss, and wellness generally with healthier expectations.

- I even have self-control.
- My willpower is my superpower.
- I'm in complete control of myself during this experience.
- I make my very own choices.
- I even have the facility to make a decision.
- I'm dedicated to achieving my goals.
- I will be able to make the simplest choice on my behalf.
- I succeed because I even have self-control.
- I'm capable of working through hardships.
- I'm dedicated to overcoming challenges.

Affirmations for Exercise

Exercise is important for healthy weight loss, but it is often challenging to plan to. Many of us struggle with motivating themselves to exercise, or to exercise enough, to require proper care of the body. If you're battling exercising, these affirmations will help drive you to figure out or motivate you to end your workout on a high note.

- I'm so excited about exercising.
- I really like moving my body.

- I'm focused and prepared to exercise.
- I'm exposure at 100%.
- Today, I will be able to have a superb workout.
- I even dare to ascertain this workout through.
- My body is becoming stronger a day.
- I really like exercising.
- Exercising is fun and exciting.
- I like becoming the simplest version of myself.

Affirmations for Healthier Habits

Your habits can play an enormous role in your wellness. From how you eat to how you sleep and the way you otherwise lookout of yourself, practices are essential. As you're employed toward losing weight and creating a healthier lifestyle, positive affirmations can assist you. With the subsequent positive affirmations, you'll make committing to your healthier habits much easier.

- It's easy on my behalf to possess healthier habits.
- I even have a simple time eating healthy food.
- I eat a daily basis.
- I select to eat healthy foods.
- I move my body daily.
- I foster healthy habits so that I can enjoy a healthy body.
- I always choose the healthy option.
- I look out of my body within the best way possible.
- I'm dedicated to taking care of my body.
- Healthy habits come naturally to me.

Affirmations for Self-Esteem

When it involves body image, self-esteem is vital. Low self-esteem is often both the explanation for an undesirable body image and, therefore, the results of one. If you are unhappy with how you look and feel, it might be because you lack the vanity to form a change; otherwise, you may feel that way due to how your health is within the times. Either way, boosting your self-esteem can now help keep you committed to your wellness goals and may improve your ability to foster a body shape and level of health that feels more desirable for you.

- I deserve a happy, healthy life and body.
- I'm a singular individual.
- Life is fun and rewarding.
- I need to have a body that helps me explore everything that life has got to offer.
- I select to be happy and healthy immediately. I like my life.
- I select to possess a pleasant experience.
- I really like and accept myself as I'm.
- I'm thriving now and forever.
- Every day I take a step toward becoming my best self.
- I need to love my body.

Affirmations for Beauty

When we are within the process of adjusting the way our bodies look, it is often difficult to recollect that you simply are beautiful in the least stages of your journey, even the parts you don't like. Having affirmations to assist you to affirm your beauty to yourself will increase your self-esteem, self-confidence, and self-worth while also helping you generally feel better about yourself.

Plus, the more beautiful you are feeling, the more likely you're to take a position in your physical wellness and appearance, meaning that you simply will become even more motivated to nourish yourself well and correctly exercise so that you'll reduce permanently.

- I'm beautiful inside and out.
- The happier I feel, the more beautiful I become.
- Once I am proud of myself, I'm beautiful.
- My skin is visible, healthy, and glowing.
- My body is gorgeous.
- I even have clean, smooth, and soft skin.
- I like admiring myself within the mirror.
- I'm a gorgeous person.
- I'm grateful for my beautiful body.
- Each day, my body becomes more beautiful.

As you continue breathing, allow these words to percolate in your mind. Feel them becoming one with who you're, together with your identity.

Feel yourself affirming that you simply are, indeed, a reliable, capable, beautiful, worthy, and fit person who will effortlessly lose the load that you simply desire to lose.

Feel yourself lovingly accepting this new, healthier version of yourself. Allow yourself to become one with this original image of you.

Believe the words and affirmations that you have repeated back to yourself and trust that they're correct—plan to believing them.

When you are ready, you'll begin to bring your awareness back to the space around you. Allow yourself to open your eyes, return to a natural breathing rhythm, and steel oneself against the day before you.

As you do, feel yourself believing in every single affirmation you heard today, and trusting that it's entirely, absolutely right.

Guided Weight Loss Sessions for Hypnosis

Losing weight with hypnosis works a bit like the other change with hypnosis will. However, it's essential to know the step by step process so that you accurately recognize what to expect during your weight loss journey with the support of hypnosis. Generally, there are about seven steps that are involved in weight loss using hypnosis.

- The initiative is once you plan to change
- The second step involves your sessions
- The third and fourth are your changed mindset and behaviors
- The fifth step involves your regressions
- The sixth is your management routines
- The seventh is your lasting change.

To give you a far better idea of what each of those parts of your journey seems like, allow us to explore them in greater detail below.

In your initiative toward achieving weight loss with hypnosis, you've got to make a decision that you desire change, which you're willing to undertake hypnosis to vary your approach to weight loss. At now, you recognize you would like to reduce, and you've got been shown the likelihood of losing weight through hypnosis. You'll end up feeling curious, hospitable, trying something new, and a touch bit skeptical about whether this is often actually getting to work for you. You'll even be feeling frustrated, overwhelmed, or maybe defeated by the shortage of success you've got seen using other weight loss methods, which can be what leads you to hunt out hypnosis within the first place. At this stage, the simplest thing you'll do is practice keeping an open and curious mind, as often this is how you'll set yourself up for fulfillment when it involves your actual hypnosis sessions.

Your sessions account for stage two of the method. Technically, you're getting to move from stage two through to step five several times over before you officially enter stage six. Your sessions are the stage where you engage in hypnosis, nothing more, and zip less. During your sessions, you would like to take care of your open mind and stay focused on how hypnosis can assist you. If you're struggling to remain open-minded or are still skeptical about how this might work, you'll consider switching from absolute confidence that it'll help to possess a curiosity about how it'd help instead.

Following your sessions, you're first getting to experience a changed mindset. Often this is where you begin to feel much more confident in your ability to reduce and in your ability to stay the load off. At first, your mindset should be shadowed by doubt, but as you still use hypnosis and see your results, you'll realize that you simply can create success with hypnosis. As these pieces of evidence started to point out up in your own life, you'll find your hypnosis sessions becoming even more powerful and even more successful.

In addition to a changed mindset, you're getting to start to ascertain modified behaviors. They'll be smaller initially, but you'll find that they increase over time until they reach the purpose where your expressions reflect precisely the lifestyle you've got been getting to have. The simplest part about these changed behaviors is that they're going not to feel forced, nor will they desire you've got had to encourage yourself to urge here: your changed mindset will make these changed behaviors incredibly easy for you to settle on. As you continue performing on your hypnosis and experiencing your changed mind, you'll find that your behavioral changes grow more significant and more effortless every single time.

Following your hypnosis and your experiences with changed mindset and behaviors, you're likely getting to experience regression periods. Regression periods are characterized by periods where you start to interact in your old mindset and behavior once more. This fact happens because you've got experienced this old mindset and behavioral patterns numerous times over that they still have deep roots in your subconscious. The more you uproot them and reinforce your new behaviors with consistent hypnosis sessions, the more success you'll have in eliminating these old behaviors and replacing them entirely with new ones. Anytime you experience the start of a regression period, you ought to put aside a while to interact during a hypnosis session to assist you in shifting your mindset back to the state that you want and wish it to be in.

Your management routines account for the sixth step, and that they inherit place after you've got adequately experienced a big and lasting change from your hypnosis practices. At now, you're not getting to got to schedule as frequent hypnosis sessions because you're experiencing such significant changes in your mindset. However, you'll still want to try to hypnosis sessions regularly to make sure that your mindset remains changed, which you are doing not revert into old patterns. Sometimes, it can take up to 3-6 months or longer with these consistent management routine hypnosis sessions to take care of your changes and stop you from experiencing a big regression in your mindset and behavior.

The final step in your hypnosis journey goes to be the step where you encounter lasting changes. At now , you're unlikely to wish to schedule hypnosis sessions any more. You ought to not got to believe hypnosis in the least to vary your mindset because you've got experienced such significant changes already, and you do not end up regressing into old behaviors. Thereupon being said, you'll find that from time to time, you would like to possess a hypnosis session to take care of your changes, particularly when an unexpected trigger may arise, which will cause you to require to regress your behaviors. These sudden changes can happen for years following your successful changes, so staying on top of them and counting on your excellent coping method of hypnosis is vital because it will prevent you from experiencing a significant regression in life.

Encourage Healthy Eating Using Hypnosis

As you undergo using hypnosis to support you with weight loss, there are a couple of ways in which you're getting to do so. One of the methods is to specialize in weight loss itself. Differently, however, is to specialize in topics surrounding weight loss. For instance, you'll use hypnosis to assist you to encourage yourself to eat healthy while also helping discourage yourself from unhealthy eating. Practical hypnosis sessions can assist you in bust cravings for foods that are getting to sabotage your success while also helping you are feeling more drawn to creating choices that are getting to assist you effectively reduce.

Many people will use hypnosis to vary their cravings, improve their metabolism, and even help themselves acquire a taste for eating healthier foods. You'll also use this to assist and encourage you to develop the motivation and energy to truly prepare healthier meals and eat them so that you're more likely to possess these healthier options available for you. If cultivating the motivation for cooking and eating healthy eating has been problematic for you, this sort of hypnosis focus is often incredibly helpful.

Using Hypnosis to Encourage Healthy Lifestyle

In addition to helping you encourage yourself to eat healthier while discouraging yourself from eating unhealthy foods, you'll also use hypnosis to assist and encourage you to form healthy lifestyle changes. This way will support you with everything from exercising more frequently to learning more active hobbies that support your wellbeing generally.

You may also use this to assist you in eliminating hobbies or experiences from your life, which will encourage unhealthy dietary habits in the first place. For instance, if you tend to scoff once you are stressed, you would possibly use hypnosis to assist you in navigating stress more effectively so that you're less likely to scoff once you are feeling stressed. If you tend to eat once you are feeling emotional or bored, you'll use hypnosis to assist you in modifying those behaviors, too.

Hypnosis is often wont to change virtually any area of your life that motivates you to eat unhealthily or otherwise neglect self-care to the purpose where you're sabotaging yourself from healthy weight loss. It truly is an incredibly versatile practice that you simply can believe, which will assist you with weight loss, also as assist you with creating a healthier lifestyle generally. With hypnosis, there are countless ways in which you'll improve the standard of your life, making it an incredibly useful practice for you to believe. You'll use hypnosis to support yourself with weight loss, also as improving your wellbeing overall.

The Right State of Mind

Find a quiet place to take a seat or lie for complete relaxation, then breathe and concentrate. Notice that the air tides in through your nostrils and the way your belly buzzes to the utmost and gently falls back to your spine as you exhale. Allow gravity to carry you securely in situ. Breathe as naturally as you'll. Don't force your breathing and notice if your breath is quick or slow and steady.

As you inhale, accept gratitude and let warmth fill your lungs. Consider the items you're grateful for. Consider something that creates you are feeling happy and peaceful. Tell yourself, "I am thankful to be alive. I'm secure and safe. I'm confident and pure." concentrate on your heart now. As you say these words to yourself, feel them deep within you. Give these statements positive energy and feed them amorously. "I love myself; I can do anything I put my mind to. I trust that my brain, body, and soul are capable of providing me with what I desire most in life."

Breathe in now and fill your mind and soul amorously and heat. Imagine as you inhale that there's a radiant light that fills your lungs before rapidly escaping your body. This light gives your patience, it gives you strength, and it provides you with the ambition and motivation to tackle the barriers that substitute your way. Exhale naturally and see as your body becomes heavier. With every breath that flows out, abandoning of negative thoughts; push those thoughts aside. You're ok, and you'll do that. You're loved. You're special. Exhale and release all of the strain that holds you back now. What people believe and what you think are two various things. Say this far, "I believe myself."

Count your breaths now. As you inhale, breathe together with your belly and count. One, two, three, four, and five. Once you are abandoning this breath, confirm it's steady and slow. Exhale, two, three, four, five. You're accepting this positive light to vibrate through your entire being. You're letting go of all the negativity that holds you back. Inhale one, two, three, four. Exhale one, two, three, four. And inhale for one, "I am happy," two, "I am strong," three, "I am kind," four, "I am brave," five, "I am driven to succeed." exhale now. You're counting your breath from one to 5 slow and steady. Positivity embraces you now; you are feeling light and in complete control. Nothing can disturb you; nothing can bring you down; you're perfect the way you're. Repeat this step until you're able to watch your thoughts flow in and out.

Bring focus to your inner thoughts now. What pops into your mind? If you've got any negative thoughts, allow them to be there as long as they need to be without judging them. Watch them, then let them go. With every in-breath, notice your thoughts enter without judgment. These thoughts are neither positive nor negative. Once you exhale, just abandoning all hostility and anger you would possibly be holding. Let it escape into the universe and inhale, one, two, three, four, five; you're accepting all honesty and trust within yourself that you simply can make it through anything.

"I am resilient. I'm beautiful. I'm a pacesetter ."

If you notice any negative thoughts, just see them and replace them with positive, self-loving thoughts.

Breaking Barriers

Make sure that you simply are during a place where you're completely comfortable and cannot be disturbed for a minimum of thirty minutes. Have the space you're inset to a comforting temperature and confirm that the lights are low. Adjust your body so that your shoulders are relaxed, your arms are lying on either side of you, and your palms face the ceiling. You would like to become as comfortable and relaxed as you'll so that your focus isn't on your body but the meditation. Gently close your eyes and take a deep breath inward until you do not inhale. Exhale slowly and steadily so that all of the air escapes your lungs. Repeat these two more times.

Notice how your mind and body are relaxing into this guided exercise now. Breathe naturally now and convey your attention to your breath. Notice because the air fills your lungs and escapes as quickly because it entered. Breathing are some things we do a day that we frequently deem granted. It's one of the various gifts that life gives us. Just be mindful of this moment you're in immediately. Don't be concerned if your mind wanders; that's natural. There are no wrong thanks to doing that. Put trust in yourself that directly, you're not performing; you do not need to be perfect.

Bring your attention to your body and your weight now. Visualize in your mind what you appear as if and check out not to judge yourself too harshly. You're who you're, regardless of what you look as if or how you are feeling that. Erase the strain and negativity from your mind; just be present with yourself immediately.

Say to yourself

"I am beautiful. I'm strong. I can do that. I will be able to reduce, and that I won't let anyone or anything substitute my way. The sole opinion I will be able to accept is what I feel and feel about myself. At this moment and in my future moments, I think that I'm beautiful just the way that I'm ."

Let your breath suck these thoughts altogether and have your mind believe everything you tell yourself as if it had been your last wish on Earth.

As you visualize your weight immediately, I might, such as you to imagine that you are at the start of a race. There are people a bit like you're competing for fulfillment.

Say to yourself

"I got this. I will be able not to hand over. I will be able to succeed, and that I will make it to the finishing line. I will be able to conquer my fears and overcome every obstacle that stands in my way."

In the background, you hear a teacher shout, "Ready, get set..." Bring your awareness to your breath again. Inhale deeply, and as you inhale, get yourself fully committed and prepared to require your initiative toward losing weight. "Go!" exhale and visualize your feet, taking that first, second, and third breakthrough. Feel the pressure of your body depress on your legs and carry you forward. You realize this is often hard, but you do not hand over. You still jog ahead. Repeat this – "I know I can, I do know I can, I do know I can. I won't hand over; I can do that ."

You are now arising to a bicycle, and as you get thereon, you are feeling the bike hold your weight. You'll not fall. Put your feet on the pedals and begin cycling. As you cycle, you continue faster and faster. Your heart is racing from the much-needed exercise. You are feeling good. Your lungs start to harm, but you push yourself as you notice the wind flying through your hair. Notice the droplets of sweat cool your skin. You bought this, and you're coming to a curve within the course now. Turn your bike and follow the trail to the finishing line. As you reminisce, you'll see people a bit like yourself competing to end, and there are a couple of behind you and a couple of before you. While exercising, take a gentle breath in and push it out forcefully. You ought to hear a pushing sound coming from your pursed lips. Inhale and say, "I got this, I won't hand over. I will be able to succeed." you're coming to the finishing line now, but the course isn't over yet. As you cross the finishing line, you get off your bike in third place. Thanks for going!

Bring your attention now to your breath. You're breathing heavily, your heart is racing, your chest hurts, but it is a euphoric feeling. You are feeling free; you broke out of the cycle and crossed the finishing line. As you're taking a glance down your body, you notice your body has become thinner. There's a scale ahead of you on the sidelines; you've lost ten pounds. the sensation you're experiencing at this very moment is breathtaking, so you would like to undertake it again. Trust that your body knows you and what to try to. Trust in yourself that you simply will get through this.

You prepare again and wait to listen to the coach. Take a deep breath specific a count of 5 . once I count, you'll start your course. Five, four, three, two, one, and go! Let loose your breath and feel your legs carry your ten pounds-lighter body. This point is a little more comfortable than the initial round. Your breath quickens, and your heart accelerates. You'll do that.

Say to yourself

"I will complete this course. I'm strong enough to overcome any barrier that stands in my way. This way is often hard, but nothing easy is worth doing. I got this."

In front of your now's a blow-up house with a good opening. You crawl through this opening and are covered by colorful plastic balls. They're flying at you from all angles, and it becomes hard to ascertain. Soon, you're swimming through these balls moving forward. You push these balls aside, and as you search, you see another opening. "I got this,"

You tell yourself

"I will make it through, and zip can stop me now." As you reach the opening, you crawl through and are entirely on your stomach. You're during a narrow hole that you simply must army-crawl through to succeed in the top. Absorb a deep breath now. Nothing scares you. Nothing can get to you. Imagine this hole the way everyone else bullied you or picked on you. You would possibly have felt small, or enclosed, singled out, or trapped.

You have complete control, and you'll do that. You're coming closer to the sunshine at the top now. Nothing can stop you. As you reach the top of the tunnel, you leap out and begin doing jumping jacks and yell to the universe, "I did it!" You beat your fears, and you conquered the darkness, but your journey isn't over yet. On the proper side of you, there is water on the table with a scale right next to it. You down the water and tread on the size. You notice your weight dropped another ten pounds. because the euphoric energy escapes you, you are feeling happy and delighted.

As you look before you, you see another course twenty feet away and, therefore, the finishing line at the top. Take a breakthrough now. Walk or jog at your own pace. You bought this. You've got faced harder challenges before, so you're getting to get through this one. Twenty steps later and you reach a potato sack, and five tires on the bottom laid call at a line. You jump into the potato sack, and while holding it up, you jump into the first tire hole. Take a deep breath in, and now the second tire hole. Exhale, jump into the third tire, now the fourth, and take some time. Inhale and jump into the ultimate tire.

As you leap out to end, exhale slowly. You'll feel your heart aching from the exercise. Pat yourself on the back; you're almost there. On the left side of the track, you notice weight balls that attach to your ankles and two five-pound dumbbells. You connect the ankle weights, devour the dumbbells in each hand, and appearance forward. The finishing line is ten steps away. Take a deep breath in. "I'm almost there, I won't give up." exhale and take your initiative. The load around your ankles was an equivalent amount of weight you carried at the start of the race. You notice what proportion of a difference this is often and never want to desire this again. Take another breakthrough and feel the sweat drip down the rear of your neck. Feel the exhaustion.

Now visualize your ideal weight. Let that be your motivation to continue. With every step, you become more and more tired. Your body becomes more and more exhausted, but you do not hand over, you retain moving forward; the finishing line just steps away now. Take a deep breath in, and there's no way you're abandoning now. You're so on the brink of your ideal weight. You've got almost accomplished your goal. You hear the people on either side of you cheer you on. Yes! You crossed the finishing line and felt that it had been all worthwhile as you step onto that scale beside you. And right before your very eyes are the numbers you've got wanted to ascertain for therefore long.

You did it! Congratulations! You're now at your ideal weight. Visualize what this seems like and absorb the thrill. Visualize what feeling you'd experience after completing your goal. Stay relaxed at this moment for as long as you'd like.

When you are ready, come to this moment. Bring your awareness to your breath. Move each finger and wiggle your toes. Feel good as you remember your visualization. You completed your goal, and you didn't hand over . that is what you'll prefer to neutralize your waking life a day. Everyone has obstacles, but you've got the willpower and now the talents to beat everyone that gets in your way. You'll open your eyes now.

Perfect Weight

"Of perfect mind and ideal weight." The terms could seem sort of fantasy to you; the sound mind and, therefore, the ideal weight. They're the realistic conditions it's possible to use as you pursue weight reduction. "Realistic?" you ask. "How can anything be 'ideal,' including my burden and my ideas about my weight?" Well, recall what we said about the facility of believing and belief. Can it serve your curiosity to desire or hope for love or money but perfection on your own? Indulge us for a few times as we clarify why you can think your mind and burden as "perfect."

Perfect weight is the weight that's ideal for you. It is the weight that's achievable and according to everything you would like and what you're able to give yourself and accept on your own. More to the purpose, your ideal weight provides you the healthy body, the body which matches effortlessly, and also the one where you're feeling great about yourself and joyful. And what're ideal thoughts? You currently have a complete thought process, and it's flawless. But there are often a couple of ideas in those typical thoughts of yours that are providing you undesirable outcomes. There is usually something you hold in your mind, possibly habits or routines, which give you adverse outcomes. However, you'll use your ideal thoughts to align your ideas to supply you precisely what you desire. You'll use your thoughts to accomplish the bodyweight you want.

In the Twinkling of an Eye Fixed

Your current body is the outcome of your ideas and beliefs. You've acted out these ideas and feelings by the way you reside, which generated your current weight. You haven't made any errors, no matter what you'll be thinking of yourself; instead, you've just experienced undesirable outcomes. These unwanted effects are an instantaneous effect of misaligned ideas and beliefs about yourself, which are your very patterns of behavior or way of life. The Self-Hypnosis Diet is all about using your ideal thoughts to align your ideas to supply you with the results you desire. You can actually use your mind to accomplish the bodyweight you want.

Now, watch the learnings have occurred in your life, which has gotten you to where you're now together with your weight. Are you able to awaken one afternoon, and there, you're using all the extra pounds? Or was it a slow accumulation with time? Or perhaps you've understood nothing else from early youth. Regardless of the situation, many factors made your body what it's today, such as:

- Food choices
- Eating customs
- The self-critic in you
- Economic history
- Emotional background
- Influence of household
- Impact of friends
- Cultural heritage

All these and several other variables were learned in your life and eventually became your beliefs, which subsequently became patterns of activity that generated your weight. We'll be more specific and notice which those aspects appear right for you in your previous years. In other words, consider what you probably did understand in your youth about eating and food.

- What sorts of grocery did your household buy?
- What meals did your parents cook, and were they typically ready?
- Do you consume food, only reception, or does one often grab fast food?
- Have you been served fresh, healthy, home-cooked foods, or did you eat mainly processed and highly processed foods, fried foods, and "junk" foods?
- What did you understand about eating mindfully?
- Have you been taught that healthful food options led to healthy bodies?
- Did anyone teach you ways you'll understand what's healthy food and what isn't?
- Were your food selections supported, which tasted or seemed great or priced less?

Examine your own socioeconomic or sociocultural roots, and see whether or not they had an impact on the way and what you learned to consume. Over thirty-five decades back, sociological research acknowledged weight issues from the working and class consistent with their intake patterns of what has been referred to as "poverty-grade foods," like hot dogs, canned meats, and processed luncheon meats.

Cultural groups even have been analyzed to know their dietary patterns and meals, like cooking with lard or ingesting a diet of high fat and fried foods, which will cause higher body fat gain. These influences can readily be accepted because they're "normal" within the group or course. Then let's take a glance at the adolescent years. During adolescence, were there any changes in your weight? As a boy, were you invited to pile more food on your plate? "Look at him, eat more! Certainly, he's getting to become an outsized guy!" (There's a telling metaphor) Or are you currently admonished to eat? When you are a budding girl, did a sensible girl take you under her wing and ask you that the marvel of menses and, therefore, the wonderment of body modifications, as an example, organic growth in body fat with the expansion of breasts and broader shoulders?

Were you conscious during puberty, wherein, unless your body improved body fat by 22 percent, it wouldn't correctly grow and make menses? Or was that "hushed up" within a clumsy improvement? It had been likely during adolescence which you heard there is a stigma regarding obese men and ladies. Spend a few minutes writing down the aspects that appear to be accurate for you in your previous years. Ponder the encounters and influences which formed your body.

In high school, the athletes at school sports have always been a wholesome weight, so are also the cheerleaders and homecoming queens. What could ancient beliefs about your popularity and self-image have formed out of the societal interactions in high school? What did you understand about physical activity, and what customs did you produce? Have you ever been introduced to physical activity as a part of a healthy lifestyle, through family or sports outings of walks or hikes? Or was the blaring TV a traditional fixture, enticing everybody to the sofa?

Next may be a question which most of the people haven't been conscious of during their evolution. As you're growing up, was the eye of self-care supported trendy clothes, makeup, and hairstyles, or on healthy food, routine physical activity, and spiritual and intellectual nourishment? What about today? Spend a few more minutes writing down the aspects that appear to be accurate for you within the past few decades. What influences and experiences shaped the ideas, which turned within the beliefs, which become a body?

After high school, you moved far away from home. Suddenly, you do not accept as true with your family's lifestyle. Did you become more conscious of your options, or did you begin eating to detach steam? If you entered into an in-depth connection, what compromises or arrangements about food and physical activity, did you share input? Most relationships develop from similar pursuits, like food preferences and eating styles. Within the end, the connection comprises eating routines and tastes, which are a consequence of compromise. Have your relationships encouraged smart food choices and healthy eating? Maybe you've experienced pregnancy. Are you able to learn the thanks to getting a wholesome pregnancy and nourish a healthy infant within you? Or did you add pounds?

After parturition, did your lifestyle assist you in recovering your healthy weight or inhibit it? Within the event that you simply were active during a league or sports matches, did your livelihood or family duties take priority and eliminate these fitness activities from your regular? Did you correct your exercise and diet? Or did the load begin to accumulate? Did an accident, injury, or illness happen that disrupted a traditional physical activity that has been supportive of a healthy weight?

It's possible to notice that how you bought and to where you're now was no accident. You heard from the parents around you and, you also collated out of the environment the way to produce food decisions. The thanks to eating, and, therefore, to taking care of yourself emotionally and physically. Whether the ideas you heard were great and healthy or not so great and not so healthy, they became your own beliefs, and eventually became you and your body because it is today. Bear in mind, you didn't do anything wrong, but you've experienced the outcomes of eating and living, which are according to your ideas and beliefs.

More than the years, what's been your answer to people and their opinions about your weight loss? bad or good? Are you able to leave and buy an incredible pair of sneakers, or did you consume more to ease the psychological distress? Maybe you even heard the latter response in your youth. Did your mom ever provide you with a plateful of food to comfort you once you felt miserable? These are learned responses, and that they are often unlearned and replaced with new answers and patterns to form your ideal weight. You ask, "Just how long does this take?" We inform you, "In the twinkle of an eye fixed ." For the minute you understand that you simply need it enough to try to anything to possess it, it's completed. You've just altered the management of highly efficient energy in you, which can be directed at deciding the way to get the result which you need: your ideal weight.

Your Perfect Mind Relearning

It isn't difficult to grasp how you bought or "heard" to weigh over your ideal weight. And it will be simple to make new decisions, to relearn new routines, and also to form new and far healthier habits. How can we learn? The simplest and most lasting learning entails repetition and practice. The most straightforward thanks to training are vital.

Pretend for a moment that you are a violinist. You're rehearsing for a grand symphony operation in NYC. Your piece includes a neighborhood of 5 pubs that's extremely hard for your fingers to perform correctly. There are two ways in which you practice. The first, which is sort of ineffective, would be to play that tough segment fast, over and over and once again, always playing the same mistakes, but trusting that your hands will play it properly

The next way is to the clinic, which can always be useful. Here, you perform the section very slowly, mindfully "teaching" your palms the thanks to maneuver, making the "muscles" ready for the acceptable moves. You are doing this steady until your palms have discovered the steps and may play the entire segment correctly and within the appropriate pace with small, if any, mindful focus.

The important thing here is that you're giving your attention to practicing correctly. By being conscious of what you're exercising, and therefore the way you're practicing it, you're studying the new patterns which are replacing the previous routines. You're practicing the action that generates your ideal weight. You, too, can create "muscle memory" by practicing mindful eating (eating slowly, chewing thoroughly, swallowing the last bite before you're taking another bite) or maybe a more cautious, slower fork-to-mouth motion. You'll even practice an entire dining design that becomes conditioned as mind-body learning or memory, which instantly becomes intuitive. Because it will become an inherent or second character, you do not get to believe doing it.

Tools for Reducing Body Weight

Stimulus Control

The skill of keeping your environments stocked healthy food choices and cleared of trigger foods that make temptation.

For many years, the man spent an intrinsic part of his life chasing down food to eat. Today during a world overloaded with food choices, food is now chasing us, and it's winning.

Fat Thinking and Stimulus Control

I always ask Shift Weight Mastery Process participants to list the environments, times of day, and trigger foods they reach for. Most of their lists aren't long, but they're explanatory!

- Cheese once I return from work—with wine!
- Crackers or chips ahead of the TV.
- Eat from my boss's candy jar within the afternoon when I'm stressed.
- Eat leftover cake within the staff room.

Nine times out of ten, when a client has had an error and increased a couple of pounds, it's because of a tempting food or a specific set of meals among the environment.

Never underestimate the facility that food— especially an interesting trigger food—has on your brain and your ability to regulate it.

Trigger foods are foods that you simply can't eat just a touch of. They tend to be a food that activates your brains got to eat more and more until the bag, box, or bowl is empty. Trigger foods also tend to be highly refined foods that contain big mouth and brain pleasers, like sugar, fat, and salt. There are exceptions to the present rule. Some people choose to spread , dried fruits, cheeses, or high-fat dairy. Any food you discover yourself circling back for or brooding about can pose a "stimulus" issue.

According to Brian Wansink, Ph.D., author of Mindless Eating, when adults are put into a state of perpetually having to decide whether or not to concede to food temptations, they get worn down and eventually concede. That's why counting on your ability to be strong and exert willpower within the presence of your favorite, fattening trigger food may be a sort of fat thinking. It just doesn't work.

Thin Thinking and Stimulus Control

Weight Masters adopt a proactive attitude with their environments instead of a defensive one. They use their minds to think on a particular level—protection. You'll cultivate thin thinking by choosing foods that are getting to be best for you in your environments and avoiding foods that challenge your weight release and maintenance.

Here are two thin thinking strategies which will make an enormous difference to your long-term weight release success:

- Stimulus-proof your environments, like your home, work, gym, car, or anywhere where you spend time and/or are susceptible to eat your trigger foods.
- Create loving boundaries together with your trigger foods.

Stimulus-Proof Your Environments

This three-part stimulus control strategy is incredibly easy in theory. Your challenge is to form it a practice.

Keep Healthy Snacks Available

You enter your front entrance after spending the last 45 minutes in traffic, and your blood glucose level is dropping as you head into the kitchen. You've got to start dinner, but as you open the fridge to tug out the salmon and salad fixings, the first things your eyes fall on are three leftover pieces of pizza. What proportion willpower does one need to assert not to stand there and erode least a couple of bites of that pizza, if not all three slices?

What if the pizza was within the back of the fridge during a covered container, and therefore the very first thing you saw was the salmon and green beans you're getting to steel oneself against dinner and a box of pea pods and cucumber slices to munch on while you cook. Because you wouldn't see the pizza, your mind isn't engaged to believe it and doesn't need to exert energy to resist it. Out of sight, out of mind, and out of mouth!

Make some extent once you shop to possess healthy snacks to succeed in for at work and reception and altogether of your environments. If you retain the healthier options upfront and simply available, your mind will stay tuned to nourishing yourself.

If a Food is Challenging You, Move It or Get and obviate It

There are a couple of ways to try to this:

- **Keep challenging food out of sight**. Creating a visible barrier between you and, therefore, the food sometimes is enough. I had a client who put a barrier between her and of the corn chips on the table at Mexican restaurants by placing the napkin holder and glasses to cover it. Put trigger foods in cupboards or drawers or within the back of the pantry so that they aren't in sight.
- **Freeze the trigger food**. This way works great for bagels, bread, cookies, and food. It removes the urge to pop some into your mouth impulsively.
- **Dispose of the food**. If the tactics still don't work, put the food within the garbage, and if you continue brooding about it, put the food within the trash on the road. That, my dear apprentice, is stimulus control. The rubbish disposal works well too. Remember, it's not a waste of cash if it saves you from pain and suffering. Avoiding the few hours of feeling bad about yourself is well worth the price of disposing of some trigger foods.

Stimulus-Proof Your Shopping

Millions of dollars are spent getting you to steer zombie-like down grocery aisles, putting the beautiful packages in your cart, and getting them through checkout stupidly about the later consequences to your body and your weight struggle. Don't be a pawn in their numbers game! Take back your power at the shop.

We often undermine our weight management by buying things for people at the grocery. Parents often use the excuse that “it’s for the youngsters .” Two more common explanations are “what if friends come over” and “it’s on sale.” Shift your mind and stay focused on what you would like from the grocery. Walk by anything that you simply know are going to be calling your name later that night. Make a shopping list and stick with it!

If your Inner Rebel says, “I need to buy frozen dessert for the youngsters,” but it’s you who finish up eating it, expire the frozen dessert. How? Take a deep Shift Breath, connect with your thin thinking Inner Coach, and ask yourself:

- If I buy this frozen dessert, what is going to happen to it?
- Is that frozen dessert getting to be calling my name all night?
- Is that frozen dessert getting to be for the youngsters or the guests? Will I find yourself watching rock bottom of the empty carton and cursing myself for falling for the old “it’s for the kids” con again?

Love yourself enough within the moment to mention “no” to the impulse. You're doing yourself an enormous favor by setting yourself free from the cravings, the food-sneaking behavior, and, therefore, the guilt after you eat it. Just walk on by. have you ever passed the frozen dessert aisle yet? Phew!

Stimulus-proofing your environments may be a potent strategy. You'll be amazed at what proportion easier weight management is when your settings are freed from the trigger foods that cause you problems.

I am not saying that you simply need to remove all the unhealthy foods or treats from your house. I'm sure many diets don't hook you. I do know that I can have bags of potato chips sitting in my cupboard for months and that I couldn't care less. Chips don't roll in the hay on behalf me so that they don't get to leave my house. However, it's a particular issue altogether once you are talking candy and gumdrops! Those sugary candies are a trigger food on behalf of me. I do know if I even have one, I also have to eat the entire bag. So, guess what? They don't are available at my house. If they are doing, my family is under orders to not let me know. What my mind doesn't realize won't stimulate it.

Creating Loving Boundaries with your Trigger Foods

Life is long, and there'll be times once you want to enjoys an enjoyable treat, including your trigger foods. How does one set your mind up for fulfillment when having that treat? Make a rule together with your Inner Coach before time about. When and the way much of a gift you're getting to enjoy. That treat isn't an option at the other time. I call this strategy, "creating a loving boundary."

Alain Dagher, Ph.D., a neurologist at Montreal's Neurological Institute, conducted a study on expectation and brain activity concerning smoking. He measured the brain activity of smokers who were kept from smoking for four hours. One group was told that after four hours, they might smoke; the different group was told they needed to still abstain from smoking for six more hours. The smokers who expected the cigarette after four hours began to point out high levels of arousal, the closer their time to smoke came.

The other smokers, who didn't expect a cigarette, showed no arousal. When the brain knows that a gift or treat won't be forthcoming, it puts its attention elsewhere. Once you create a choice about something, and you're clear that boundary, it helps your mind say "no" comfortably.

Here's the way to roll in the hay step by step.

- Identify the trigger food. This way could be easy; it's the one you can't stop eating!
- Think of what one serving would be both in amount and calories. Confirm it allows you to remain within your Calorie allow Weight Release.
- Think of an environment during which it'd be safe to eat one serving. This environment is one that you simply haven't had a stimulus control issue in.
- Create a limit on how often you would possibly enjoy you trigger food during this setting. Creating a limit keeps you from overindulging or abusing the boundary.

For example, say your trigger food is a frozen dessert. If you didn't stop eating the frozen dessert until the carton is empty, our stimulus control strategy would be to stay frozen dessert out of your house. But what if you would like to be ready to enjoy its creamy goodness every once during a while? You'll create a replacement loving boundary with a frozen dessert.

For example, a loving boundary for frozen dessert could be “Once every week, and I can have a scoop of my favorite at the frozen dessert parlor.”

You are giving yourself something you enjoy but during a moderate and measured way outside your environment. You'll even search the frozen dessert calories online and see that one scoop of rocky road is 170 calories. You'll make it work calorically for you on the day you have it, too. You've got the frozen dessert but still, remain within your Calorie allow Weight Release.

My Loving Cake Boundary

The frosting was my drug of choice once I struggled with my weight. At one wedding, I went back for five pieces of bride cake. Of course, I had to stay face. I didn’t want the server to think that I used to be an out-of-control cake fiend. I told him that I used to be bringing the additional slices to others at my table. Little did he know that the others at my table were my Inner Rebel and her wild friends partying on cake deep inside me!

As I started my journey to weight mastery, I created a healthy and loving boundary around the cake that works on behalf of me still. I tell myself, “Cake and frosting on behalf of me isn't an option unless it’s my birthday or the birthday of anyone in my immediate family.”

This fundamental rule around the cake may be a perfect fit for me. For every family member’s birthday, I will be able to make a cake and have an exquisite piece with extra icing. In my inner rule system, the cake isn't an option unless it's my birthday or my husband's and children's birthdays.

Create Your Trigger Food Loving Boundary Exercise

Take a flash to fill in your trigger foods and make a loving boundary.

- Stimulus-proof your environments by removing the trigger foods that tempt you and having healthy choices available, once you aren't falling victim to high-calorie foods in your situation, it's much easier to remain consistently on target with weight release.
- Bringing healthy food into your environments and having them available for meals and snacks is different to make sure your situation is about up to assist you in succeeding.
- Create loving mental boundaries around your favorite trigger foods so that you'll have them in your life occasionally but in a controlled way. Knowing your trigger foods and creating a masterful relationship with them puts you responsible.
- Stimulus control is a crucial skill not just for releasing weight but also for long-term weight management.

APPRENTICE PAUSE: have you ever felt protective of somebody or something? Perhaps you've got cared for a little child or a pet? It's quite an intense feeling, right? Why is it that when it involves your self-care and weight, you don't step in to guard yourself? Now that you simply understand the skill of stimulus control, you'll be your protector, bringing a replacement level of self-protection to your life within the way you're taking care of yourself and, therefore, the environments you reside in.

Weight Loss Hypnosis

To start this hypnosis, confirm that you simply are during a comfortable position. Don't attempt to do that once you are driving and wait to try to it publicly, like on a bus or a plane. You are doing not skills your body might react, so it's best if you're focused on doing this reception while on your couch, or perhaps as you're falling asleep. Remove all other distractions and focus only on staying comfortable. Focus only on your breathing and hear the subsequent directions as you begin to fall under a relaxed state.

For this hypnosis, you're getting to visualize what's waiting ahead of you. Let the thoughts flow through your mind as if they're your own.

Everything that we are getting to discuss during this motivation is about you, and only you. We are getting to begin with "I" statements because these are affirmations. These are the thoughts you would like to urge into your head to rewire the way that you only are thinking towards something more positive and healthier.

I am inhaling and that I can feel myself fill with life because the air enters my body. Because it comes, I count one, two, three, four, and five. Because it exists, I count six, seven, eight, nine, ten. Counting my breath helps me to manage it. When my breathing is regulated, everything else in my body is going to be also. These processes are reliable, and that I understand that my body is capable of anything.

I have begun to concentrate on the items that I'm eating to assist me in reducing. Within the past, I used to be unhealthier and that I made poor decisions for my body. This way has led me to where I have gained weight, and now, I feel unhappy with the person who I even have become.

I have tried to reduce it within the past. I even have considered eating foods that are bad on my behalf and that I may need also considered some unhealthy dieting methods, like crash dieting or harmful pills.

I did this because I used to be taught to hate my body. I wanted to punish myself for the shape that I had found myself in after making more unhealthy choices. I made unhealthy decisions to undertake and reduce, not that specialize in my psychological state within the process.

These unhealthy choices led me to an area of negative thinking. I feel bad thoughts about my body, which only makes it harder on behalf of me to reduce.

At this moment, I'm getting to stop this negative thinking. I will be able not to be focused on hurting or punishing myself anymore.

The only thing I care about is ensuring that I'm a healthy person. I'm focused when it involves my health and, therefore, the foods that I'm putting into my body. I care about the wealthy , but I care even more about feeling better.

I am uninterested in trying a new diet after a new diet. Each new thing I discover, I buy small hope, but it fails. It doesn't fail due to the meal plan, but due to my mindset. I buy frightened of what is going to happen once I fail, so I'd not even try within the beginning.

I am not getting to allow myself to think like this anymore. I'm only getting to be focused on positive thinking and a healthy mindset to assist within the achievement of my goals. I don't want to urge stuck within the same thinking pattern for the remainder of my life. I deserve better. I deserve entirely just hating my body. I need to be happy from the within, which will start to point out on the surface.

I am always surprised at how hard my body works because it consistently exceeds my expectations. Once I am sick, I'm wondering if I will be able ever to feel better, but my body does most of the add fighting things off. I'm ready to achieve great things with my body, and therefore the only reason I'd have fallen off my healthy lifestyle path within the past is that I did not see that initially.

Going forward, I'm getting to be focused on seeing the fantastic things that I'm capable of. I'm only curious about tracking the items that I even have done. I'm not focused on the topics that I'm still waiting to accomplish. I'm grounded within the "now," because that's the sole thing that matters to me during this weight loss journey.

I am centered with my body, and I'm determined to urge it to the right place. I'm not getting to try anything harmful to reduce. Instead, I'm getting to work with my body, not against it. I'm getting to use the tools that are the foremost helpful in ensuring that I reduce successfully, so I don't need to worry about it returning on later in life.

I am taking a positive path towards getting the items that I desire. I felt like weight loss took goodbye before. Often this is because I used to be tracking my progress multiple times each day. Within the past, if I didn't see results within a few days, then I might think that something wasn't right.

I understand now that this was just a mentality that was taught to me. My body works much faster than I'm ready to see, but I wont to only measure it by the items that were happening on the surface.

Moving forward, I'm only focused on measuring progress with how good I feel. Accepting this mentality alone makes me feel better already. once I am clearly focused on ensuring that my psychological state is that the most vital, then everything else seems such a lot easier.

The reason weight-loss felt love it took goodbye within the past was because I used to be impatient. I understand how time works now and that I realize that I can't track things as closely as I want to. Within a month, I will be able to see far more progress than what's seen during a day, and that I understand the difference now.

I am understanding of how I want to twiddle my thumbs, and the way this mentality will help me to reduce rapidly. If I buy too impatient, I will be able to attempt to rush a process that takes time, and it'll only make it feel longer within the end.

I am not getting to give my attention to fast weight loss.

I am getting to ignore the size.

I will only specialize in numbers during a long-term sense, like monthly weigh-ins.

I am getting to be the foremost concerned with how I'm feeling mentally.

If I ignore how I feel mentally, then this may only hold me back further and keep me within the place that I'm already trying so desperately to urge out of.

I am not getting to fight against my body anymore. I'm only getting to confirm that I'm using its natural processes to reduce. Once I am often patient, it'll make the load loss feel much faster.

I am getting to keep track of my weight loss reasonably, and I'm getting to drop the unrealistic expectations that I've created for myself.

I am getting to be compassionate to myself during this process.

I understand that I will be able to make some mistakes.

I have the motivation and encouragement needed within myself to form sure that I don't let these mistakes become defining moments in my life.

Each time I feel as if I even have slipped far away from a goal, I will be able to remember that it's up to me to urge back on target from an area of determination and dedication.

I am getting to be forgiving of myself for my natural urges and need to follow old habits.

I am getting to be more reliable than the person who I used to be within the past, but I also remember that they're still strong themselves.

I am focused only on living a healthy lifestyle and losing weight rapidly. I understand that thanks to making this process fast is to stay to it. There are not any shortcuts or quick fixes. This way is often a process that's getting to be a lifelong journey, but that doesn't mean I can't still see results within a comparatively close time-frame.

I understand that being patient and sticking this diet out is what's getting to help me reduce the quickest.

I accept the very fact that I cannot rush this process and need to take it because it comes. My body knows what it's doing and that I trust that it's the facility to form up for the items that I cannot control. I'm getting to encourage my body to reduce through keto and fasting, but it'll still be up to my body what proportion weight I will be able to lose and at what pace.

I will not compare my body to others anymore. I'm only focused on myself and that I know that I even have all the facilities needed to seek out success.

As I continue during this hypnosis, I'm reminded of where I'm now and where I will be able to be going next. I'm getting to count to 10, and once I reach ten, I will be able to be out of the meditation and either drifting to sleep or back within the world where I'm more focused and prepared to lose the load. My breathing remains regulated and can still plan the hypnosis has ended. One, two, three, four, five, six, seven, eight, nine, ten.

Meditation

Today's world is simply so fast-paced that it seems like we've no time to hamper, relax, and be calm.

Even once we continue the holiday, we take over the office and add our heads, worrying about subsequent committee meetings, a disgruntled client, or where the next deal comes from.

We think we're happy and calm, but within our minds, there are many hidden stresses, fears, worries, and thoughts going deep. Once we don't take time to relax and quiet the inner noise consciously and intentionally, tension will build up and inevitably affect the standard of our lives, and the way we affect people around us.

It needn't be like this. Meditation practice will allow us to settle down and obtain still. It helps our mind to urge concentrated and relax, helping us to deal with all the everyday stresses of a busy life.

Not Just a spiritual Act.

People typically classify meditation as being purely for religious or spiritual activities. Although many religions are correct to form reflection a part of their religious practice, it's not merely a mental activity alone. But more and more people that aren't religious accept meditation practice.

If you are feeling like life is getting a touch too hectic and leaving you stressed, then slowing down, calming, and relaxing would be an excellent time. Meditation will assist you in achieving a relaxed state you would like to ease your mind and free from stress.

Meditation Advantages

Still, wondered why people are meditating? Which difference, which value does it bring back their lives? I used to be at a coffee point in my life once I started meditating and crying about the loss of my friend. I started meditating on my counselor's suggestions as to how to assist and ease my worries and continue my wellbeing and core strength building cycle.

A lot of individuals have various reasons to meditate. Once you are contemplating, what was your reason to meditate? To an outsider, if you meditate, what they see you are doing is sit down, maybe cross-legged on the ground, watching some extent within the distance or sit together with your eyes closed.

How does this, practicing meditation, influence your state of mind? Yet most of my students in yoga and meditation swear that meditation for quarter-hour each day is that the neatest thing they will do to offer them the strength, motivation, and compassion they have to try to whatever they have.

Meditation is a few mental activities that have significant health benefits both for the mind and, therefore, the body. Meditation can help relax the mind, establish a more concentrated state, and enhance the functioning of the brain.

Medical evidence suggests that meditation practice appears to elicit A level of physiological relaxation: decreases in vital signs, slower heartbeats, and faster breathing, and other biochemical improvements can occur also.

- Meditation reduces the consequences of many chronic illnesses, like a heart condition, cancer, and diabetes.
- It helps and soothes chronic pain, anxiety, and migraine.
- Meditation helps improve the role of the system and also prevents binge eating.
- The asthma attacks offer considerable relief.
- Reduces lactate within the blood, minimizing depression and anxiety.
- Meditation has been documented to also help in lowering cholesterol.
- Reduces muscle tension, and therefore the system is relaxed.
- It assists in building self-confidence.
- It helps monitoring aggressive mind.
- Increases synchronization between brain waves.
- Removing unhealthy habits helps.
- Assists in the creation of intuition, imagination, and concentration.
- It improves the power to recollect and enhances memory retention.
- Enhances sleep habits and assists in eradicating insomnia.

Meditation is the process of thought intensely for a short time or relaxing one's mind. This fact will be wiped out silence or with the help of singing and is completed for a spread of reasons, ranging among religious or spiritual motives to how to induce relaxation.

Meditation has, in recent years, grown in popularity in our modern, eventful world as to how to alleviate stress. It's also emerged scientific evidence that meditation is often a valuable tool within the fight against chronic diseases, including depression, a heart condition, and chronic pain.

This ancient custom has many various aspects to it.

If you're curious about trying meditation but do not know where to start, here's another list of sorts of practices:

Breaking the trance: the two athletes (runner within the hypnotic state and idol) were taken back to their forum, and therefore the athlete returned to rest on the bank before either awakening secure and refreshed or drifting off to sleep and awakening afterward feeling refreshed, relaxed and efficient.

Having a recording that takes you thru these stages is often an accurate idea because you'll hear it and do not got to believe recalling the things. You'll use it before bedtime if you've got trouble sleeping and fall asleep to sleep afterward. If you would like to be a touch more sophisticated, you'll also help to feature some background music.

I hope you've got enjoyed this chapter in which you'll find the suggestions useful. Hopefully, it all is sensible, but please get in-tuned if you've got any questions, and we'll do our greatest to elucidate and help.

Training your mind takes time and practice, so work with it and provides it time. It's almost like physical training to urge stronger as you recognize and obtain won't to new, more useful ideas and feelings. Good luck, and have fun!

How Can I Remain Motivated to Lose Weight?

The most critical aspect of making constant and virtually infinite inspiration is linked with all the explanations you would like to lose weight.

Confine mind the broader sense of weight loss for you, like your health needs or how it can positively affect you each day, and therefore the people around you, like your family and shut friends.

Specialize in clear, observable, achievable, timely, and practical objectives. Make short but attainable goals first to seek out enjoyment and fulfillment in constant progress towards achieving long-term goals of weight loss.

Have a clear, rational mind of not being too easy or too hard on yourself to succeed in the objectives by keeping the arrogance and frustrations going distant.

Find people around you with an equivalent drive as you are doing, and you're always encouraged and challenged to continue pushing for similar goals.

When you can keep these continually in mind, you'll find that you simply will feel more motivated and determined to figure through obstacles and circumstances toward achieving your long-term goals.

Methods of meditation

Conscious Meditation

It is easy to urge trapped during a loop of spinning thoughts – beginning to believe a laundry list of activities to try, ruminating about past events, or potentially future situations – and practicing mindfulness may help. Yet, what exactly is attention? It is often described as a psychological state that needs to be fully working on "the now" so that, without judgment, you'll understand and acknowledge your thoughts, feelings, and sensations.

Mindfulness Meditation

Mindfulness meditation may be a sort of mental preparation that helps you to hamper thoughts of running, abandoning of anger, and relax both your mind and body. Mindfulness methods can vary, but a meditation on mindfulness generally involves breathing exercise, imagination, body and mind awareness, and relaxation of the muscle and organ. Practicing meditation with mindfulness doesn't require props or planning (no need for candles, essential oils, or mantras, unless you enjoy it). To urge going, all you would like maybe a comfortable sitting spot, three to 5 minutes of spare time, and an attitude that's freed from judgment.

Mindfulness meditation is the method of getting your thoughts fully present. Knowledge involves being mindful of where we are and what we do, and not being too sensitive to what's happening around us.

One can do reflective meditation anywhere. Some people wish to sit during a quiet spot, close their eyes, and specialize in their respiration. But at every stage of the day, even when driving to figure or doing chores, you'll prefer to be conscious.

You track your thoughts and feelings while practicing mindfulness meditation but allow them to move without judgment.

Transcendental Meditation

Transcendental meditation is an important technique whereby an individually defined rhythm, like a word, sound, or short phrase, is repeated during a particular way. It's exercised twice per day for 20 minutes while sitting comfortably on the brink of the eyes.

The hope is that this system will allow you to settle into a deep state of relaxation to realize inner peace without attention or effort.

Directed Meditation

Directed meditation, often also mentioned as guided imagery or visualization may be a meditation technique during which you create mental images or scenarios that you simply find calming.

Guided meditation is among the foremost standard methods of meditation employed a day by many people. During this post, we'll explore guided meditation and the way to try it.

In the purest form, guided meditation may be a sort of meditation where the individual is guided on every step of his daily practice. Someone directs you right from the primary level of sitting during a meditative pose to the ultimate phase of completing the meditation. What occurs is that in meditation, an educator or mentor provides step-by-step guidance about what to try to. It's an ancient method of conveying directions for meditation to pupils. In older times, this system has been wont to teach meditation during a group. Nowadays, because of technological development, we do not need a guru's physical presence to steer us in meditation. We will hear a master's direct guidance using pre-recorded CDs or DVDs and conduct our meditation practice. Within the absence of any meditation master professional CDs / DVDs, you'll record the instructions of guided meditation from a book in your voice then play them afterward.

Furthermore, if anyone doesn't have the potential of a voice recorder or a DVD player, during a session, he may ask his friends or relatives to talk about the written meditation instructions orally. This way, we will use the advantage of guided meditation but with none technological assistance.

However, I still believe that the utilization of a pre-recorded CD or DVD for guided meditation is that the best way for guided meditation because it removes the necessity for an individual to be physically present near you to read the instructions. It also allows you to cash in of controlled meditation, even when you're alone.

Guided instructions for meditation are often of varied varieties counting on the methods the teacher imparts. A number of the foremost collective meditation techniques utilized in guided meditation are Vipassana. This meditation involves visualization of the cycle of breathing, visual imagination, mantra recitation, a meditation on dancing, a meditation on prayer and meditation on mindfulness, etc. the simplest thanks to using guided meditation is to concentrate to a master's live guidance. If this is often not feasible, then the second-best option is to record in your voice the written instructions of meditation then hear it in your meditation practice.

Usually, this phase is directed by a guide or instructor, thus "driven." it's also recommended that you simply use as many senses as possible, like a scent, sounds, and textures, to elicit calmness in your relaxing region.

Vipassana Meditation

Vipassana meditation is an ancient sort of Indian meditation that suggests seeing things as they're. Quite 2,500 years ago, it had been taught in India. Conscious meditation movement has origins during this practice within us.

The purpose of meditation with vipassana is self-transformation through the examination of oneself. This way is often accomplished to make a deep connection between mind and body by careful attention to the sensations within the body, the sustained interconnectedness results in a cheerful account, crammed with love and compassion.

Vipassana is typically taught during a 10-day course during this tradition, and other people are expected to follow a group of rules all the time, also as for abstaining from all intoxicants, telling lies, cheating, sexual intercourse, and killing any animals.

Loving Meditation on Compassion (Metta Meditation)

Metta meditation also called meditation on loving-kindness, is that the practice of guiding good wishes towards others. Those that practice reciting similar words and phrases will elicit warm-hearted sentiments. This way is often commonly found also in meditation on mindfulness and vipassana.

It's usually wiped out a pleasing, relaxed position while sitting. After a couple of deep breathes, you slowly and steadily repeat the following words. "Just let me be happy. May I be fine. Let me be free. May I be calm and at ease". After a period of guiding this loving-kindness to yourself, you'll begin to imagine a loved one or friend who has supported you and repeat the mantra, this point replacing " I " with" you." As you continue the meditation, you'll bring back mind other members of your family, friends, neighbors, or people in your life. Practitioners are often encouraged to think about individuals who are having trouble with them.

Finally, you finish the meditation with the quality mantra: "Let every being be happy everywhere"—a meditation on the Chakra.

Chakra is an ancient Sanskrit term that will be traced back to India and translates into a "cycle." The chakras ask the energy and spiritual force centers within the body. It's believed there'll be seven chakras. Every Chakra is during a different part of the body, and every one of them features a corresponding color.

Chakra meditation consists of relaxation techniques that aim to bring balance and well-being to the chakras. Any of those techniques provides the visual depiction of any chakra within the body and, therefore, the corresponding light. Some people can like better to light incense or use crystals, which are color-coded for every Chakra to assist them to focus during meditation.

Meditation Yoga. The yoga practice has its roots in ancient India. There is a right sort of yoga classes and designs, but all include performing a series of postures and guided breathing exercises designed to encourage flexibility and relax the mind.

The poses require balance and a spotlight, and practitioners are encouraged to concentrate less on distractions and remain more at the instant.

Which meditation style you select to undertake depends on several factors. Once you have ill health and are new yoga, tell your doctor what method would be right for you.

Ways to Promote Meditation into Your Life

Treat yourself to ice cream? Are you stuck within the motorway? A lover in wait? Here's the way to make these moments a meditation.

Which one considers harder: in sleep, taming your monkey mind, or doing overtime only to take a seat still every day? Either way, fear not: by merely integrating meditation into your daily activities, you'll quickly reach a relaxed state of mind.

- Do this you would like to try to. If it's a hiking, walking, cooking, or painting, while we concentrate wholeheartedly on our favorite things, time stands still. Mysteriously, our stream of emotions, stories, and dramas fall away. Submerge yourself during this one fantastic thing, and do not attend to those pings! Then keep an eye fixed on your feelings. Calmer, then? Feeling happier? Congratulations — you've just completed a meditation on the influence of this moment. That's so simple.
- Nurture nature yourself. Life doesn't sort of a popular dietary supplement, with people hiking a day happily. And almost anytime you go outside, you'll quickly practice meditation. As you adapt to the first rhythms of nature, your breath and thoughts hamper to match the gentle march of mother nature.
- Only making yourself like your ten-year-old self and observing the clouds overhead will transmute stress. Extra credit if you think about heart types blowing down the shadows.
- Wait, not, meditate! You meet a lover, and she or he is delayed — again. Seek a smartphone meditation rather than dalliance tweeting and texting. Indeed, there's an application for that! Plug your earbuds, and you're all of a sudden, engaged during a 10-minute session that's oh-so-soothing. By the time you're done, bet you, your friend

arrives — which you welcome her with a warm embrace rather than the "late-again" eye-roll.

- Time to fly. If you're caught in traffic, now isn't necessarily the time to "be one together with your fellow riders" and surrender blissfully. You would like a serene diversion. Try a mantra meditation set to make super chill music (I am a serious DJ drez fan) or invent your own ("I am love, I'm light") and obtain lost as you walk down the lane.
- Think with pillows. You'll turn sluggishness into a sublime meditation once you have a wee little bit of resistance to roll out of bed within the morning — plus, you get to remain a touch longer! Lie still, and watch your scarcely conscious feelings. Once we bear witness, "I don't need to travel to work" becomes "I see struggle — and I am fine thereupon ." bonus points for adding a purpose to your day — sort of a decision to embrace your emotions or a love offer to friends and family.
- Eat your favorite food, drop-dead. Step into the kitchen together with your oh-so-spiritual self and scoop a little helping of frozen dessert or anything tickles your buds. I'm going with cherry Garcia from ben & jerry, so work with me: consider lifting this funny little mound on your lips. Consider the temperature, taste, and smell as cherry and chocolate bits gradually slip down your throat. This ancient tradition of mindful eating is both an important rite of contemplation and an incredible way of expressing appreciation for our abundance. Ben & Jerry: namaste!
- Meditation, meditation, and yoga, and more. Truth: Whether you're trying to touch your toes or improve your handstand, the one reason we're doing yoga is going to the super-end-

of-class climax moment once we drop into a meditation savasana. It's the physical poses that allow us to urge into that dark, still space in our minds. Regardless of what degree or lineage you practice, all postures cause a state of meditation that's all-spacious.

Daily Meditations and Habits

Now I'm close to taking you on a journey of visual imagery and relaxation to a far-off place. Enjoying vibrant and compelling images, you'll hear powerful and definite statements that will endorse many feel-good affirmations, which will improve your perception of yourself and improve your overall wellbeing.

We tend to show food whenever we are stressed in life. When problems overwhelm us, most folks tend to stress and eat, and then we experience a cycle of guilt and regret. In time, this cycle can impact how we feel about ourselves.

During this guided meditation, you'll remember the way to feel good and understand your connection to food. During times of stress, you'll study letting go of tension and to experience all that's natural and instinctive.

The experience of this guided meditation is going to be enhanced if you discover yourself a cushy and ventilated spot.

Ensure that there's no disturbance from anything or anyone for thirty minutes.

You need to settle on an edge to lie or even sit comfortably for the duration of this exercise. It's a realistic idea at this point to unplug or mute your phone.

Now, you would like to shut your eyes and steel oneself against a deep sense of relaxation and wellbeing. Remember that this is often some time, and embrace the chance to flee from the stressful world you reside in. You'll now relinquish all the unhealthy habits and learn to spice up your guiding force.

At this particular moment, there's nothing that you simply got to worry about. You're asleep, and you're safe. You'll allow the tensions of the day to dissipate so that you'll connect with your inner self. Together with your eyes closes, breathe deeply and slowly through your nose then exhale through your mouth. Once you inhale, you're taking all that's good and positive about this world into your body, and once you breathe, you're letting go of all tensions and unnecessary fears.

Now, inhale again. Inhale slowly through your nose to the count of 4.

One, two, three, and 4.

With your lungs now filled with oxygen, hold your breath for 2 seconds.

One and two.

And now exhale slowly through your mouth. You would like to exhale to the count of 4.

One, two, three, and 4.

When you inhale, you'll slowly feel your diaphragm expand once you feel the air enter your lungs. Inhale until you feel like your lungs are filled with air.

Strive to regulate the exhalation of air and confirm that you simply steadily exhale you would like to continue this cycle of rhythmic breathing.

Inhale to the count for four.

Hold your breath for a count of two.

Exhale your breath to the count of 4.

You can resume breathing normally, and you'll feel all the strain in your body slowly dissipate.

Acknowledge that your body is now beginning to feel more relaxed. Your arms and legs will start to feel heavier.

Relax the strain in your lower back, middle-back, and your upper back. We frequently tend to store tension in our shoulders. Learn to release it. Once you are abandoning the strain you are feeling in your body, you'll feel your body relax.

Elongate your neck so that there's space between your ears and shoulders. Once you slowly elongate your neck, you'll feel the mattress you're lying on or the chair that you quietly are sitting on support your back.

Now, scan your body and check if there are any areas of tension left. If you feel that there are some, then you would like to tighten the muscles in those areas and abandoning deliberately. Once you are doing this, you'll feel your body relax. You'll feel the strain leaving your body.

Now, you would like to travel into a state of deep meditation.

To do this, you would like to continue the rhythmic breathing exercise.

Imagine that you simply are now standing during a beautiful meadow with soft rays of sunlight falling on you.

You can see an arched doorway that's carved into a rising cliff.

Your surroundings look quite peaceful, and you are feeling good.

You can see golden sandy beaches behind you and azure blue skies above you.

Now, you're slowly making you thanks the arched doorway. The door is within your reach; the wood feels warm under your fingers. As you trail your fingers across the door, you'll feel a way of pleasure and wonder as you imagine what lies behind the door.

To enter, you would like to stay your mind hospitable the wonders that lie ahead. Reach out and slowly turn the handle of the door.

As you emerge, you'll see a lush and delightful, bright-green rainforest.

The air feels fresh and pleasant under the cover, and therefore the welcome change from the sun-drenched beach a couple of moments ago.

Take a deep breath then exhale to embrace this sense of peace.

As you begin to steer forward, you notice a trail that leads through this beautiful rainforest.

As you search, you'll see the glimpses of a gorgeous blue that's speckled with soft, cotton-like clouds.

Continue scanning the sky all around you.

You are surrounded by majestic mahogany trees that reach up tall towards the zenith.

You marvel at the dark brown bark of the trees that seems to possess a delightful sweet odor.

Space is restricted here, but you're grateful for the narrow trail that leads you thru this place of natural wonder.

You can hear the melodious chirping of birds all around you.

It seems like the forest has to wake up around you.

All of this appeals to your senses, and you're ready to experience nature in its pristine form.

Consider if you strip back your own life and are to measure more naturally what proportion better will you are feeling.

Only a little percent of sunlight can penetrate onto the ground of this rainforest. So, you progress further call at the wilderness, and you'll see the flashes of exotic blue butterflies dancing around you.

You can hear the melodic sound of running water within the distance, and you are feeling compelled to maneuver towards it.

As you're taking within the wonder of the beautiful nature all around you, you progress towards the larger expanse of the forest area that results in a weak stream of water.

There are natural stepping-stones that lead you to a pool of water that appears crystal clear. Green plants surround the pool of water.

You walk closer to the pool, and you notice plants with colorful berries all around.

There are several fruit-bearing plants, and everything looks rich, exotic, and tempting.

You take a bite of those delicious berries, and you'll feel a burst of flavors.

The berries taste delicious, and you'll feel this deliciousness because it makes its way right down to your stomach.

Your body feels energized.

Some stones are present around and across the water, and as you walk, you begin to become one with nature.

You notice carefully carved out steps higher within the rocks, and you begin to climb.

The climb is sort of easy, and it feels almost effortless.

You feel an exquisite stretching in your muscles once you grip the rocks for balance.

There is no fear of falling.

As you grip the rocks and make your high, you are feeling slimmer, stronger, and toned.

You feel exactly how you would like to explore and the way you would like to be.

You pull yourself up higher and better . you're slowly progressing towards the cover.

You can feel the air become purer.

You start to inhale pure oxygen and abandoning of any tensions you're holding onto.

Your 'normal' looks like it's miles away.

You consider how good you are feeling at this moment.

You still make your way towards the cover.

You don't need to fear the peak since it's safe, and you can't fall.

You don't feel tired or exhausted. During this world, you are feeling fit, healthy, and knowledge of an abundance of energy. You're determined to urge to the highest and see the view from the highest of the cover.

Imagine walking up through these steps until you reach the ultimate stage and you reach the top of your journey.

You reach an outsized platform that overlooks the tops of the trees.

Directly across from you, there's a rock face with water cascading down. The water is frothing abreast of its way down the rocks, and therefore the sight is mesmerizing.

You can reach up and touch the clouds. You'll feel the clouds around you.

The sky looks beautiful.

Visualize these pleasant sensations that course through your body during this instance.

You experience a way of relaxation. Every inch of your being feels good.

Take this moment and visualize yourself stretching.

Stretch up high and feel the wonderful sensation as you elongate your spine. Now, keep your back flat and move forwards and down. Allow your body to relax forward. Imagine the incredible stretch you'll feel within the ends of your legs- there's no pain, just a joyful sensation of movement. Your spine starts to relax, from your lower back through to your neck as you lift your arms. Your neck and your head relax as you lie on the mossy platform.

Keep your arms behind your head and your elbows wired. Engage your core muscles and check out to lift your shoulder and your head towards the clouds above.

Visualize yourself lifting and interesting those core muscles while you attract your stomach and tighten your abdomen. All of this causes you to feel so good.

Now start to relax once more.

Start to consider your breathing. Inhale as you open up your chest and exhale slowly.

It is time that you simply start to feel good about the person you're. It's time to feel content and embrace pure inner peace. Here during this rainforest, you're liberal to explore and be the person who you would like to be.

Let go of any unhealthy eating habits, and it's time to be kind to your body and to nurture and protect your body.

Repeat these affirmations to yourself and believe each word.

Believe in the message and, therefore, the power these words need to change your life.

I will change my perception of my body.

I recognize my self-worth.

I will change my eating habits so that I see my food as fuel and nutrients instead of food.

I will exchange binge eating for breathing techniques and guided visualization.

I will start exercising and changing how I look and feel.

I will create an activity diary and plan the way to embrace exercise.

I can face my inner fears and make the required positive changes.

Sit quietly for a flash and let these affirmations become a neighborhood of you.

It is time to feel positive about your life.

It is time to face any weight issues head-on.

You have the facility to try to so.

At any time, you'll return to the present rainforest and knowledge of the wonders of nature. You'll find your inner strength and inspiration during this shelter.

You are centered, and you keep the sensation of peace and wonder.

Enjoy the instant and, therefore, the feeling of harmony that you simply experience.

Breathe in then out.

Retain your sense of peace and your desire to nurture your body.

Breathe in and out.

You will change your association with food.

Breathe in and out.

Slowly open your eyes on the count of three.

One, two, and three.

Now, you're back in your reality.

Stretch your body slowly and still take deep breaths.

Realize how good you are feeling during this moment.

Remember your desire to enhance your fitness and your wellbeing.

Return to the present shelter of yours whenever you would like to enhance your health.

You can use this system anytime you are feeling tensed or nervous. Whenever you are feeling stressed, rather than reaching for a packet of chips or the other food, you'll do this simple exercise to calm your mind. You'll breathe thanks to a stress-free life.

Cleansing Relaxation Meditation

This meditation is all about focusing on becoming relaxed and cleansed. One of the best ways to achieve this kind of feeling is through the use of music.

Make sure that you are somewhere comfortable. You need to be in a peaceful and distraction-free zone in which you can close your eyes and focus on nothing but feeling the air come in and leave your body.

One of the reasons why we struggle to lose weight is that we are so stressed. Stress can lead to stress-eating and cause your body to hold onto weight that it does not need. Worse, it can alter your hormonal levels.

You are focused now on reducing stress because this means that it will be easier for you to lose weight. There is nothing else that you are concerned about other than becoming more relaxed.

You are centered; you are focused. You are at this moment; you are prepared for whatever might come your way. You are not concerned with anything other than relaxing and becoming more peaceful.

Feel it as the music beats to a rhythm. There is a slight beat, no matter what it is that is being played. Everyone who listens to this will find a different meaning to the tunes. Everyone who partakes in the process of listening to cleansing music does so for various reasons.

It will always help everyone to relax. Though we all have different things that we use this music for, it still helps us to become more and more at peace. Calmer and calmer. More and more relaxed.

Start to focus on your breathing now. Breathe along with the music. Count for at least five while you are breathing in and then five as you are breathing out.

Breathe in for one, two, three, four, and five. Breathe out for six, seven, eight, nine, and 10. Feel as you breathe in how the music enters your body. Your body is like a musical song as well. Your heart is like the drumbeat that is always pounding.

Your brain is like the conductor that tells everything how it should sound. Your blood, your muscles, and your organs – they make up the rest of the instruments. Your body is a beautiful chorus, and you are a melody traveling through life.

You are a perfect being, relaxed, calm, and at peace, and you are one with the earth. You are one with the music. You start to feel it come in and out of your body.

This music can change the way you feel, and this music is in control of your emotions. It will affect the way you operate.

It is helping you to feel better and more relaxed. It is bringing you closer and closer to being at peace. It is bringing you closer and closer to being centered and focused.

You are feeling lighter and lighter, and the stress is drifting away. As soon as you start to let go of stress, you will begin to release yourself from the heavyweights that are keeping you back. The more focused you are on your breathing pattern, the easier it is for you to feel relaxed. The quicker you focus on peace, the more weight you will lose.

Each time you let go of stress, you are letting go of some of your weight. Every time you focus on being more at peace, you are feeling healthier and healthier.

You feel it as the music spreads to every part of your body. It starts in your mind. It stimulates your brain so that you are focused on relaxing and nothing else at that moment.

It soothes your heart. It reminds you that you are not alone. It makes you feel better, and that spreads everywhere else.

The music keeps you motivated. It keeps you cleansed.

Cleansing is an important part of your weight-loss journey. Your body is always working to clean itself. Your body is focused on how it can rid itself of toxins and bring in the things that are good for it. Your breathing is one way that your body is consistently working to cleanse itself.

Your body is always cycling in new air and getting rid of the old. It does the same thing with food as well. It brings in new minerals and nutrients and gets rid of the toxins that it does not need. You drink water to help cleanse your body. It is always working on its own to keep you as purified as possible.

The cleansing processes help you to feel more at peace. You feel like a new person, and you are constantly given second chances. It is never too late to start over.

You are feeling your body become more and more cleansed now. Then you are feeling lighter and lighter, more relaxed. You are becoming a new person. You are starting over. You are starting fresh. You are relaxed. You are focused. You are at peace.

As we count down from 20, you will exit this mediation. Continue listening to cleansing music to bring in the peace that you need to lose weight and maintain it. It will be easier to lose more weight when you manage to focus on cleansing.

Twenty, 19, 18, 17, 16, 15, 14, 13, 12, 11, 10, nine, eight, seven, six, five, four, three, two, one.

Dealing with Food Addiction

Until now, you've got been taking note of multiple reasons for weight gain. Some may say that overeating causes weight gain; some may believe that it's due to hormonal issues. Some may say that the lazy routine is that the explanation for obesity. We cannot deny them. All of them are correct. But if you dig deeper, you'll find causes of most problems in your head, including overeating and other purposes that are mentioned.

How does a food addict's brain differ from a naturally lean female brain? This section describes the most characteristics of the differences within the mind, especially in food addicts.

We are crazy about food. -We usually force us to eat. -We need more menu to be full. -We often suffer from hunger. -We respond more strongly to food references. -Emotional imbalance causes brain hunger in us.

Functional Resonance Imaging (fMRI) uses the magnetic properties of blood to work out which area of the brain is most active when a topic experience a specific event. Neuroscientists can measure brain activity when food addicts are exposed to food labels, eat delicious foods, or eat certain foods. "It's like training," explains Dr. Ashley Gerhardt. "When you train a specific muscle, blood flows into that area. The brain seems to be working a similar way, and you'll track which area of the brain receives the first blood."

fMRI consistently shows that the convergence zone for sensory information is that the prefrontal cortex, associated with reward stimuli, particularly primary reinforcement factors like food. To elucidate the neurobiological mechanisms by which weight, mood, and age affect the appetite response, Dr. Gerhardt presented healthy, average weight, obese adolescent and adult women with color photographs of foods with different fat content and caloric density while undergoing fMRI (high reward vs. low reward). She shows that food-addicted women skilled highly rewarded foods within the same way drug addicts answer drugs.

Dr. Bart Hoebel, originally from Princeton University, he was one among the primary to review a mouse for sugar addiction. He showed that each drop of sweet they swallowed increased the amount of dopamine. Almost like human addicts, Hoebel's rat sugar developed a hypersensitive dopamine receptor that was hyperresponsive to a spread of medicine, and its changes were long-lasting. Even after a month of self-discipline, the taste of sugar stimulates the rat to become addicted.

In a similar study, in Birmingham at the University of Alabama, Dr. Mary Boggiano found out that a food attack in rats elicits an equivalent pleasing receptor within the brain that drug addicts are stimulated once they ingest drugs. Dr. Boggiano's oleo-conjugated rats have long-term changes in endogenous opioids within the brain and become abnormally aware of delicious food.

And if this chou tastes nearly as good as sex, it's no coincidence. The dopamine reward system is that the way we feel good and is related to obsessive gambling, drug abuse, and sex. Food satisfaction results from several equivalent neural signals and pathways that regulate orgasm. As a result, many neuroscientists have begun to record that obesity, eating disorders, and even healthy appetite resemble addiction. "Repeating dopamine over and over is what drug abuse does," says Dr. Hoebel. "This causes you to wonder if food may have addictive properties.

Food gives you a discreet physiological response within the same way that drug consumption gives you an enormous response," says psychiatrist Walter H. Kaye, director of the Eating Disorders Program at the University of California, San Diego. The drug takes over the food reward. "Drugs are addictive because they open the way for appetite.

Like other drug therapies, food therapy is an effort to realize the dopamine levels required by all addicts. During a 1954 study identifying amusement centers, two McGill University researchers, Dr. James Olds and Dr. Peter Milner, documented the consequences of dopamine. During this study, rats were ready to push the bar to electrically stimulate the amusement center or push the bar for food. Dr. Olds and Dr. Milner said electrical stimulation of rats to an amusement center is more rewarding than eating. The experience was so satisfying that the hungry rat ignored the food for pleasure the electrical impulse from the entertainment facility gave her. Some rats stimulated the brain quite 2,000 times an hour for twenty-four consecutive hours. Most mice died on an empty stomach.

Heroin and cocaine addicts also happen to ditch eating and lose tons of weight while taking the drug. This fact explains why you get dopamine fixes from other sources. The primary stage of affection, all the activities that we discover so enjoyable, we don't eat much and forget to eat! Poisoning is high dopamine, not food. If this mechanism fails, we find yourself eating an excessive amount of food, hooked into repairing dopamine.

So, that's how you overeat. You are doing not eat because you wish it, but you eat because you're compelled to consume. Now we'll check out sorts of overeating.

Types of Overeating

Based on the rationale, the habit of overeating is often divided into two types:

- Obsessive overeating
- Compulsive overeating

Obsessive Overeating

Dr. Gearhardt, a scholarship recipient at the Yale University Rudd Center for Food Policy and Obesity Center, conducted a neurobiological study and documented similarities in how the brain responds to drugs and delicious foods. Like drug addicts, food addicts struggle with increasing desires, encourage them to dine in response to food alerts, and should check out of control when eating delicious food. Even as one drink sends alcohol to a bend, some biscuits also can cause seizures.

"The results of this study back the idea that increasing expectations for food may partially cause forced diets," said

Gearhardt. Counting on the expected food intake, participants with higher levels of food obsession showed more significant activity within the parts of the brain alleged to create the motivation and urge to eat, but with suppression of inhibiting mechanism during impulses. Liable for consumption, which showed less activity within the area of responsibility.

Gene Jack Wang, MD, director of drugs at the Brookhaven National Laboratory in Upton, NY, and Dr. Nora Volkow, director of the 'National Institute on substance abuse,' said this was just a perspective on human imaging studies and grilled chicken. The smell of hamburgers and pizza releases dopamine into the brain. This food stimulus significantly increased dopamine levels within the minds of gluttons, but not in non-gluttons. the quantity released correlates with the intensity of one's desire for food for an extended time, the subjective impression "I search for it."

"This is how our brain controls our desires," said Dr. Wang, many food addicts feel weak in their ability to regulate when and the way much they eat. The wall unit contains the striatum, a neighborhood of the emotional brain that contributes to motivation, and therefore the neurotransmitter dopamine, which controls the search for pleasure and produces pleasure. "Now we're not just talking about balancing the energy state," he says. "We are discussing human psychology," said Wang.

Compulsive Overeating

The ventral striatum of the brain is best known for its role in motor pathway planning and coordination. Still, it's also involved during a sort of other cognitive processes, including executive functions like memory. In humans, the striatum is activated by reward-related stimuli, but also by an aversive, novel, unexpected, or intense triggers; and, therefore, the symptoms related to such events. Once you see the brain sort of a train, the striatum on the ventral side is that the accelerator.

When food enters the physical body, it stimulates the amusement center, which increases the flow of dopamine. When overeating becomes standard behavior, three things happen:

- The reward system is kidnapped,
- Neuroplastic changes occur,
- Serotonin and GABA (inhibitor) neurotransmitters involved within the "brake system" are reduced.

Food addiction confuses entertainment centers. It's more like when brakes of a train break down, and runaway trains eventually get down the tracks. All are accelerators, no brakes. Forced or compulsive overeating is like this.

Why We Overeat?

Eating is one of our biological needs and is ensured by the enjoyment we feel once we eat. But as soon as we got hooked on food, like long-term alcoholics became ready to drink everyone under the table, and as drug addicts needed more and more medicine, we develop a higher tolerance to food. All sorts of addiction require increasingly addictive substances to succeed in dopamine levels. Chronically strong drinkers have few signs of addiction, with high blood alcohol levels, which are either impossible or fatal to non-drinkers. Tolerance facilitates the consumption of overconsumption of alcohol, which results in future physical addiction. Similarly, the addict's brain needs more food to supply the amounts of dopamine that are related to normal high-grade foods.

Men who believe web pornography during the study are one of the foremost moving samples of forgiveness. As soon as a person completely relies on this type of dopamine fixation, he reports that he's unable to be agitated or satisfied during intercourse with a true woman. They take months to travel without an X-rated website and endure severe withdrawal symptoms before they will regain the enjoyment of interacting with a true woman.

In 2001, alongside his colleagues, Dr. Volkow, including Dr. Wang, a Ph.D., obtained brain scans of overweight and normal-weight volunteers to review the enumeration of dopamine receptors. Dr. Wang noticed that overweight people had lesser dopamine receptors-the, the more obese they were, the less these important receptors that they had (the brains of addicts). He says the brains of overweight people and drug addicts are strikingly similar: "Both have fewer dopamine receptors than normal subjects."

All addicts are trying to find an answer, but if we become more immune to our drugs, in our case, eating food, a little amount of non-delicious food, reduces the feeling of joy and results in the underproduction of dopamine. Something stagnates within the process of the generation of dopamine within the brain. Genetic damage is named polymorphism. If one among the genes required for the dopamine process may be a polymorphed, it'll appear in those certain people with prominent symptoms.

Again, dopamine may be a neurotransmitter produced by our brain once we enjoy eating. Once you enjoy a delicious salad, pot, or slice of pizza, roll in the hay because your mind produces a healthy amount of dopamine. So, overeating is forcing us to repair dopamine.

The misconception that fat women have more fun while eating than thin women is flawed. The fMRI again shows that a healthy brain produces far more dopamine than the mind of a food poisoner. Food addiction has an equivalent adverse effect as the other addiction. The addicts developed greater tolerance for the drugs of choice, and low dopamine levels mean less experience with pleasure. Therefore, most addicts consume a large amount of food once they want to realize the expected amount of delight. This fact is one of the apparent and measurable differences between a naturally lean female brain and an obese female brain.

This phenomenon explains why we absurdly act once we don't reach the food levels that cause the assembly of dopamine enough to experience a pleasure.

Food poisoners suffer overwhelming hunger within the presence of food. Overeating obsessively and compulsively, when not hungry, are more vulnerable to smells and a robust desire to eat, even after a full meal. Researchers call this phenomenon "external food hypersensitivity." British Medical Research Centre presents a study during which brain scans have shown how this food susceptibility affects people's diets.

Researchers Andrew Calder, Luca Passamonti, Ph.D., and James Rowe, Ph.D., sought to seek out why some people tend to overeat. Within the Journal of neuroscience (January 2011), brain scans of the human were presented to point out three sets of images of participants (delicious food, boring food, and irrelevant photos of other subjects). Their response was then recorded.

"People who appear to be more interested in food have different connections in their brains, " said obesity expert Marc Andre Cornier, MD, an endocrinologist at the University of Colorado, who has nothing to try to with this study.

Dr. Gearhardt von Yale discovered that: "Addictive people respond physiologically, psychologically, and behaviorally to triggers, like advertising. Delicious foods are always available and highly marketed today. Within the food environment, it's important that food-related symptoms can cause pathological reactions." Like drug addicts, food addicts have increased appetite and appetite in response to flood warnings. You'll feel that you simply are out of control once you eat delicious food, and you lose your strength while eating, and therefore the feeling that you simply cannot help yourself becomes dominant. This way is often beat stark contrast to naturally lean women who don't even know that this type of fighting is feasible.

Emotional imbalance causes hunger. Take a positive person, whose strongest allergies are everything that influences his optimism, and who eats whenever his energy state is low. The strain is relieved by eating. Also, for uncomfortable feelings, difficult situations, and difficult people, everything out of the sunny temperature results in a visit to the kitchen.

When we are hooked into overeating, our brains are programmed to use food to temporarily relieve anxiety, frustration, stress, depression, agitation, and discomfort with dopamine modification. The longer you employ food to enhance your mood, the more likely it's that you only are going to be related to relief from feeling sick with addictive substances. Once we experience life's ups and downs with low tolerance, our primary coping mechanism is dopamine modification. Emotional imbalance results in excessive episodes of eating.

Starting Mindful Eating

You certainly already know: Naturally lean women have several properties that cause a healthy relationship with food:

- They only eat once they are physically hungry.
- They take the time to organize a healthy meal.
- They specialize in their eating experience and, if possible, eat them silently.
- If possible, they dine in a pleasant place.
- They enjoy the food.
- They only take a little bite.
- They often put the dishes down.
- They wholly and slowly chew the food.
- They breathe consciously before chewing the food.
- If food loses its taste, they stop eating immediately.

What is the idea of most of those habits? Eat wholeheartedly. I used to be always intrigued when Naturally Thin Women used this phrase. But what's mindful eating? I wanted to understand what they did once they ate carefully. Use four TCB steps to revive these 10 NATURALLY THIN WOMEN'S properties. Let's check them out:

- Recognize old patterns step
- Interrupt the old pattern step
- Perform NTW operation steps mindfully and with complete attention
- Measure progress and knowledge success

Now we'll undergo these properties of naturally thin women during a detailed manner:

Recognizing Physical Hunger

Step 1: Identify Starvation for the Situation

Five sorts of triggers instigate current overeating programming. All of them are explained below:

Social Incentives: They eat to avoid feelings of inadequacy or to share a standard experience, hoping that it connects them to the others. There's scientific evidence that we eat quite a lot once we dine in a social environment.

Sensual Trigger: Eat for Opportunity, Eat Donuts at Work, Advertise Food for Food on TV, or travel by the Bakery. I didn't feel the necessity to nourish my body, but I had the chance to experience joy and suddenly felt hungry. In these cases, the will to eat is a chance to experience the learned response, a pleasure to external triggers. We weren't hungry until we saw the visual food.

The motivation for thought is: Eating as a result of internal dialogue that condemns oneself. We offend ourselves, and ironically, succumbing to overeating usually reprimands us for lack of willpower.

Physiological trigger: Eating in response to a physical effect (e.g., headache or other pain).

Emotional triggers are: Eating in response to boredom, stress, fatigue, tension, depression, anger, fear, and loneliness. These triggers are as simple as a scarcity of cognition within the body (I need a physical break) or as complex as suppressed emotions (I'm a member of a toxic family).

Step 2: Break the Obsession

My brain is crazy about food. I'm hungry and wired to form me feel obsessive about responding to food. This way is often my current wiring that uses food counting on different situational triggers.

Step 3: Name and Address Your Actual Needs

Depending on things, you've got the choice of the way to respond effectively to the trigger.

Social Trigger: to satisfy the will to attach with others, I can try a couple of small bites and rave about the food. Even better, you'll start an exciting conversation about something aside from the menu.

TCB Answer: this is often not a pang of physical hunger. This way is often my desire to adapt to society.

Sensual Trigger: Recognizing my usual reaction to the visual appeal of food. I admit I wasn't hungry before I saw the menu. We must assume that this is often not physical hunger; it's an automatic response to the unexpected.

TCB Answer: this is often not a pang of physical hunger. This way is often my Pavlov's response to a highly charged stimulus.

I would like to enjoy the pleasure that food presents. If I eat this sweet, I will be able to feel better.

Motivation: Recognizing the standard reaction to negative thoughts, pain, and discomfort. Ending emotional stress may be a normal human reaction. I even have alternative and meaningful ways to affect feelings of inadequacy.

TCB Answer: this is often not a pang of physical hunger. Eating may be away on behalf of me to settle down and the way I weaken my painful thoughts. I even have the tools or can get the assistance I want to affect the painful dialogue inside.

Physiological triggers: There are simpler tools (medication as needed) to affect physical complaints.

TCB Answer: this is often not a pang of physical hunger. This way is often a learned reaction to physical illness.

Emotional triggers: you'll identify what triggers your emotional hunger and prefer to act effectively.

TCB Answer: this is often not physical hunger. That's my standard coping mechanism and current wiring.

Step 4: Measure Progress

What about after performing steps 1-3? The scales within the Step 4-Measures of Progress and knowledge of the Success section assist you in measuring progress as you adopt individual characteristics. The more you practice, the better it'll be.

Is it possible for you to reply to every signal appropriately? If the solution is not any, what's your stress level? Have you got to reduce stress first? What are the wise decisions to satisfy your actual needs?

Take Time to Prepare A Healthy Meal

Home cooking has many advantages because it is a sort of mindfulness. You choose top quality and nutritious ingredients. Confine mind that grocery stores are supported cheap fats and cheap carbohydrates, not your nutritional value. You're controlling where your calories come from: they are available from trans fats, additional sugars, well! They make sure that there are not any flavor enhancers like MSG or other brain-disrupting substances. As mentioned earlier, the internet effect of those addictive substances is that you simply eat more. Creating a healthy diet is expressing your love for yourself and your family. It is a creative achievement. Economize with this exciting vacation-like activity in Tahiti, Paris, and, therefore, the Galapagos Islands. You'll spend the maximum amount of time as you would like . you'll come up with several tricks and shortcuts to save lots of time within the kitchen. It's honest and to recover your cooking skills. It only takes a couple of hours to revive the master chef inside. At the same time, to travel somewhere to select up food. Clarify the facts, go there, park, get food, eat there, or take it home. Consistent with the middle for Disease Control (CDC), cases of quite 76,000,000 people that suffered from gastrointestinal disorder annually thanks to bacteria, viruses, and parasites that cause food contamination.

Think about it; you've got to eat carefully. the sole area that affects 95% of this possibility is that the quality of the food you eat. If you do not know who cooks or exactly what ingredients they use, are they cheap trans-fat oils, much extra sodium, extra sugar? How are you able to manage yourself?

Sitting in Beauty

Establish a natural and delightful environment, especially if you eat alone. Albeit you're hungry, it can take a couple of minutes to succeed in a beautiful setting. If you do not have the time, are during a hurry, and need to eat directly from the fridge, this is often an enormous sign that you're usually absorbed in foods that are perceived as high levels of hysteria. This fact might feel irresistible while restoring a naturally lean female neural network. This way heals the "hungry brain," so it's important to calm before eating. There are several ways to scale back high levels of hysteria like deep breathing, meditation, journaling, active jogging, and anything that seems personally effective in reaching an area of peace. Remember to live your progress. Are you able to found out the table without fear? If not, could you be known to identify the explanation for anxiety and address it?

Eating Experience

In a culture that emphasizes multitasking, eating may be a secondary activity. We don't combine food with the nutrition of our bodies. Consumption is what we do without attention while doing more meaningful work.

Have you automatically turned off your car radio while trying to find a replacement address? I instinctively know that removing a voice stimulus increases your ability to specialize in finding its address. Silence also allows us to concentrate only on food and to be fully present for a dining experience. Watching TV, interacting with computers, talking on the phone, reading books, and doing other activities isn't a supplement to a careful diet. Mindful meals require indiscriminate attention, so it is a good way to overeat.

If you've got resistance to silent hoods, rewiring can assist you in recognizing that you simply ate for the first time once you had another activity. It's a custom that has been cultivated for several years. You rarely eat the most focus.

When you sit quietly and eat, you'll hear inner conversations like the way to enjoy the meal and subtle messages from the body once you are satisfied. If turning off competing stimuli creates fear, inhale, and note the explanation for the anxiety.

If you're dining together with your family, invite them to participate in the careful process of eating. Trying to show off as many distractions as you'll during your meal is best than overeating during multitasking. Discuss your senses and taste of food. Slow food doesn't need to be extreme. Nevertheless, it's a realistic idea to remind the family that eating isn't a race. Encourage the family to chew on every slice of food, examining the taste, texture, and odor intimately. Ask them about their feelings, thank them for collecting brownie points, and thank them for his or her blessings and share their meals with their families.

Remember to live your progress: how does one feel in silence after a meal? Are you able to eliminate all distractions and eat quietly without fear? Is practicing this property easier to eat silently?

Enjoy Your Meal

Of course, the skinny women have an indoor dialogue of appreciation and appreciation and joy: "This is delicious. And it saturates. Shoveling food not only misses every bite of taste, but the wall unit is in situ. You will need more food to satisfy gourmet merchants because you are not inspired by it.

We acknowledge that this resistance to internal dialogue is that the current practice of not attending for the pleasure of eating. Usually, our conversation feeds on something aside from our body, so it's more relevant to issues, concerns, and current to-do lists.

If you pay 100% attention to eating and luxuriate in eating carefully, you'll find that the restoration of NATURALLY THIN WOMEN'S wiring is approaching.

Remember to live your progress. How does one feel after allowing an indoor dialogue about the pleasure of eating? Does one enjoy this conversation without fear? If the solution is not any, what are the obstacles to achieving this trait?

Small Bites

If you overeat food, you'll burn more calories and knowledge an equivalent amount of delight. We must recognize that we've made significant efforts within the past. The wise action is to eat some meals with a little spoon sort of a wheel while we learn to require smaller bites. However, once you measure progress during this area, it's essential to form the inside track larger. The rationale is that if you're taking a little bit simply because the spoon is low, the neural network won't be restored, and you're entirely hooked into the tool.

Don’t forget to see your progress. How does it desire after eating the entire meal with just a couple of bites? How was your fear? Did you experience the fun with such a little morsel? Did you've got to hit the kitchen and obtain a more oversized spoon? Or did you only start eating together with your fingers?

Fork Down

Whatever your fork or tableware is placed during a bite, you're encouraged to eat wholeheartedly. We can enjoy every bite, every bite, every subtlety, every spice, every texture. Eating is foreplay, not a race. It is a sensual experience. Arashi defeats the aim.

Remember to live your progress: how does one feel after eating an entire meal and placing a fork during a bite? What's your fear level? Would you wish to enjoy the delicacy of food?

Chew Slowly and Thoroughly

For many obsessive eaters, diet represents an answer for drug users. The faster you'll move the shovel, the quicker you'll rise. Unfortunately, this behavior results in total calorie burn and shortens the feeling of delight. We attempt to raise our dopamine levels as soon as possible! We've been doing this for an extended time, so biting slowly and slowly are often anxious.

The digestion begins with the first bite, causes the discharge of saliva, disinfects food, and smooths the thanks to the stomach. As we bit, the brain releases neurotransmitters that tell the hypothalamus that we are full. Wholly and slowly chewing will remove even the slightest aroma and increase your enjoyment.

Remember to live your progress. How does one feel after biting slowly? What was your fear? Are you able to enjoy the slowdown without fear?

Breathing

After swallowing, breathing three times will reconnect with the body. If you favor, it's a sort of palate wash. Readjust for subsequent bite sensual experience. This way is often also a chance to assist us in determining if we are full.

Remember to live your progress. Does one breathe three times during one bite with one meal? Did you notice that your anxiety is growing? Did you enjoy your meal?

Experience Fullness

If you eat it carefully, you will be full if you lose taste! Against this, they're trying to find salt, ketchup, mayo, mustard, sugar, or barbecue sauces as overeaters. It's something you'll regain a cushy experience and "enjoy" your food. Additives are an effort to nullify the intelligence that tells you that you simply have enough.

I've certainly heard the recommendation to attend 20 minutes for your brain to catch up together with your ecstasy. But once we erode piranha speed, we consume tons of food. We do not skills to attend. Until then, everything was invisible. Besides, our brain isn't too slow! By listening to when food loses its initial appeal, we will instantly know when it's full.

Note that the start of this process feels strange. After all, we are wont to consuming everything on the plate. For several folks, discard food is extremely difficult because our conditioning to eat everything on the plate is rooted. A useful gizmo is to see excess food as fat in your favorite body parts. Your taste will tell this part that is ok, and every one overconsumption turns into fat.

Also, understand that we are familiar with stomach congestion and no food consumption. Initially, this is often done mechanically, but if you repeat this a couple of times, you get the particular saturation. Besides, regaining confidence within the palate signal feels free, as you did not get to experience the severity of a clogged sensation after a meal. The energy satisfaction after eating, instead of lethargy or immobility, regains your sense of freedom.

Remember to live your progress. Are you able to say "it was great" and "I'm full" without having to stuff myself? Are you ready to recognize the abundance?

Fitness Strategies

Exercise Regularly

Exercise is sweet for human health in some ways, no matter what you select to try to.

Although the DASH diet focuses on food choices, there's no denying that regular and varied exercise represents a crucial component of a healthy lifestyle and one which will confer additional benefits. For those of you who are ranging from a situation , you ought to know that any exercise is best than none, which there's absolutely nothing wrong with starting slow and easing into a more rigorous routine.

With that being said, the CDC identifies moderate-intensity aerobic activity that totals 120 to 150 minutes weekly, together with two additional weekly days of muscular resistance training, as a perfect combination to confer numerous health benefits to adults. Per the CDC, these benefits include the following:

- **Better weight management**: When combined with dietary modification, regular physical activity plays a task in supporting or enhancing weight-management efforts. Regular exercise may be a good way to expend calories on top of any dietary changes you'll be making on this program.
- **Reduced risk for cardiovascular disease**: a discount in vital signs may be a well-recognized advantage of regular

physical activity, which ultimately contributes to a reduced risk of disorder.

- **Reduced risk of type 2 diabetes**: Regular physical activity is understood to enhance blood sugar control and insulin sensitivity.
- **Improved mood**: Regular physical activity is related to improvements in mood and reductions in anxiety due to the way during which exercise positively influences the biochemistry of the human brain by releasing hormones and affecting neurotransmitters.
- **Better sleep**: those that exercise more regularly tend to sleep better than those that don't, which can be partially due to the reductions in stress and anxiety that always occur in those that exercise regularly.
- **Stronger bones and muscles**: Combining cardiovascular and resistance training confers serious benefits to both your bones and your muscles, which keep your body working at a high level as you age.
- **A longer lifetime**: those that exercise regularly tend to enjoy a lower risk of chronic disease and an extended life span.

As you'll see within the 28-day plan, your recommended exercise totals are going to be met by exercising four out of seven days every week. The exercise days are going to be choppy as follows: All four of the active days will include aerobics for a half-hour . As a beginner, I encourage you to start slowly and build up to four days. Two of the four active days also will include strength training. Rock bottom line is that you simply don't need to exercise for hours every day to enjoy the health benefits of physical activity. Our goal with this plan is to form the health benefits of exercise as accessible and attainable as possible for those that are ready and willing to offer it a try. Before we get to the great stuff, though, there's still tons of wisdom to be shared about getting the foremost out of your workouts.

Getting the Foremost Out of Your Workouts

Just as with healthy eating strategies, there are certain essential things to stay in mind about a physical activity that will help support your long-term success. Let's take a glance at a couple of important considerations which will assist you in getting the foremost out of your workouts:

Rest days: albeit we haven't even started, I'm getting to preach the importance of excellent rest. Don't forget that you only are participating during this journey to enhance your health for the future, not to burn yourself call at 28 days. Although a number of you with more experience with exercise may feel confident going above and beyond, my best advice for the bulk of these reading is to concentrate on your body and take days off to attenuate the risk of injury and burnout.

Stretching life: Stretching may be a good way to stop injury and keep you pain-free both during workouts and in daily. Whether it's a planned activity after an exercise or through additional means like yoga, stretching is useful in some ways.

Enjoyment: there's no right or wrong sort of exercise. You're being provided a various plan that emphasizes the spread of different cardiovascular and resistance training exercises. If there are certain activities within these groups that you simply don't enjoy, it's okay not to do them. Your ability to stay with regular physical activity within the future will depend upon finding a method of exercise that you simply enjoy.

Your limits: Physical activity is sweet for you, and it should be fun, too. It's up to you to stay it that way. While it's important to challenge yourself, don't risk injury by taking things too far too fast.

Your progress: Although this is often not an absolute requirement, a number of you reading may find joy and fulfillment through tracking your exercise progress and striving toward an extended duration, more repetitions, and so on. If you're the sort who enjoys a competitive edge, it's going to be fun to seek out a buddy to exercise and progress with.

Warm-ups: Last but never least, your exercise routine will benefit greatly from a correct warm-up routine, which incorporates starting slowly or doing exercises almost like those included in your workout, but at a lower intensity.

Set A Routine

The exercise a part of the DASH plan was developed with CDC exercise recommendations in mind to support your best health. For some, the 28-day routine could seem sort of a lot; for others, it's going not to appear to be that much. If we glance at any exercise routine from a general perspective, there are a minimum of three broad categories to remember.

Strength training: This involves utilizing your muscles against some sort of counterweight, which can be your own body or dumbbells. These sorts of activities alter your resting rate by supporting the event of muscle while also strengthening your bones.

Aerobic exercise: Also referred to as cardiovascular activity, these are the quintessential exercises like jogging or running that involves getting your body moving and getting your pulse up.

Mobility, flexibility, and balance: Stretching after workouts or maybe devoting your exercise time on within the future"> at some point every week to stretching or yoga may be an excellent way to take care of mobility and stop injury in the future.

This routine recommends involving a mixture of both cardiovascular and resistance training.

You will be given a good array of options to settle on from to accommodate a various exercise routine.

My best recommendation is to choose the kinds of exercises that provide a balance between enjoyment and challenge. Remember that the advantages of physical activity are to be enjoyed well beyond just your 28-day plan, and therefore the best thanks to making sure that is that the case is selecting movements you truly enjoy. My final recommendation during this regard is also to include some sort of stretching either after your workouts or on a day of rest.

Cardio and Weight Exercises

In addition to a spread of various cardiovascular exercise options, the strength-training options you'll be provided are divided into four distinct categories: core, lower body, upper body, and full body. Per your sample routine, a perfect strength workout will include one exercise from each of those categories:

Cardio

Brisk walking: this is often mainly walking at a pace beyond your regular walking rate for a purpose beyond just getting from point A to point B.

Jogging: This is often the intermediary stage between brisk walking and running and may be used as an accompaniment to either exercise, counting on your fitness level.

Running: The quintessential and maybe most well-recognized cardiovascular exercise.

Jumping jacks: Although half-hour straight of jumping jacks could also be impractical, they're an honest exercise to the different activities on this list.

Dancing: those that have a background in dancing may enjoy using it to their advantage, but anyone can place on their favorite songs and dance like nobody is watching.

Jump rope: Own a jump rope? Why not use it as a part of your cardiovascular workout? It's fun, thanks to getting your cardio in.

Other options (equipment permitting): Activities like rowing, swimming and water aerobics, biking, and using elliptical and stair climbing machines are often great ways to exercise.

Your goal, to satisfy the CDC guidelines, is going to figure up to a complete half-hour of cardiovascular activity per workout session. You'll use a mixture of the exercises listed. I suggest that beginners should start with brisk walking or jogging—whatever action you're most comfortable with.

Core

Plank: The plank may be a classic core exercise that focuses on the stability and strength of the muscles within the abdominal and surrounding areas. Engage your buttocks, press your forearms into the bottom, and hold for 60 seconds. Beginners may start with a 15- to 30-second hold and work their high.

Side plank: Another core classic and a plank variation that focuses more on the oblique muscles on either side of your central abdominals. Keep the buttocks tight and stop your torso from sagging to urge the foremost out of this exercise.

Woodchopper: a rather more dynamic movement that works the rotational functionality of your core and mimics chopping a log of wood. You'll start with little to no weight until you are feeling comfortable and progress from there. Start the move with feet shoulder-width apart, back straight, and slightly crouched. If you're using weight, hold it with both hands next to the surface of either thigh, twist to the side, and lift the load across and upward, keeping your arms straight and turning your torso such, you finish up with the weight above your opposite shoulder.

Lower Body

Goblet squat: Start your stance with feet slightly wider than shoulder-width and a dumbbell held tightly with both hands ahead of your chest. Sit back to a squat, hinging at both the knee and, therefore, the hip, and lower your legs until they're parallel to the bottom. Push up through your heels to the starting position and repeat. Use a chair to squat onto if you don't feel comfortable.

Dumbbell walking lunge: Start upright with a dumbbell in each hand and feet in your usual standing position. Breakthrough with one leg and sink until your back knee is simply above the bottom. Remain upright and make sure the front knee doesn't bend over the toes. Erupt the heel of the front foot and breakthrough and thru with your rear foot. Start with no weights, and add weight as you are feeling comfortable.

Romanian deadlift: Unlike the squat and lunge, the Romanian deadlift puts the primary emphasis on the rear muscles of the legs (hamstrings). Substitute an identical starting position to walking lunges. Still, this point you'll hinge at the hips and push your buttocks and hip backward while naturally lowering the dumbbells ahead of you. Squeeze your buttocks on the ascent back to the starting position. You'll also do that exercise on one leg to enhance balance and increase core activation—however, and you'll get to use lighter weights.

Upper Body

Push-ups: These are the last word body-weight exercise and maybe done almost anywhere. You'll want to line up together with your hands just beyond shoulder width, keeping your body during a line and always engaging your core as you ascend and descend, without letting your elbows flare. Those that struggle to perform push-ups consecutively can start by showing them on their knees or maybe against a wall if regular push-ups sound like an excessive amount of.

Dumbbell shoulder press: an excellent exercise for upper-body and shoulder strength. Bring a pair of dumbbells to ear level, palms forward, and straighten your arms overhead.

Full Body

Mountain climbers: On your hands and feet, keep your body during a line, together with your abdominal and buttocks muscles engaged, almost like the highest position of a push-up. Rapidly alternate pulling your knees into your chest while keeping your core tight. Continue during this left, right, left, right rhythm as if you're replicating a running motion.

Always attempt to keep your spine during a straight line.

Push press: this is often primarily a mixture move incorporating a partial squat and a dumbbell shoulder press. Employing a weight that you simply are comfortable with, stand feet slightly beyond shoulder width, with light dumbbells held during a pressing position. Descend for a squat to a depth you are feeling pleased with, and on the ascent simultaneously push the dumbbells overhead.

Burpee (advanced/optional): this is often a classic full-body exercise that's essentially a dynamic combination of a push-up, a squat, and a jump. This particular exercise is extremely effective but could also be challenging for a few and will be utilized only by those that feel comfortable. The correct sequencing of the movement involves ranging from a standing position before lowering into a squat, placing your hands on the ground, and jumping backward to land on the balls of your feet while keeping your core strong. Jump back to your hands and jump again into the air, reaching your palms upward.

Stay Hydrated

Proper hydration by beverage is a crucial habit that supports healthiness and weight management. Caloric drinks with minimal nutrients, like soda, became an increasingly common source of calories in our population, and replacing such beverages with plain beverages may be a valuable step to require better health. Using natural flavors sort of a splash of lemon may be a great way to transition from drinking sweetened beverages to plain water.

It is recommended that ladies drink about 11 cups each day, and men drink about 14 cups each day. Confine mind that this includes fluid from both foods and beverages, not just water. Particular sorts of food, especially fruit and certain vegetables, have very high-water contents.

Beverages like coffee, tea, and soda water also count toward your daily totals. Drinking enough water also will help prevent constipation and work alongside the fiber from your diet to stay your bowels working effectively.

Stress Management

There are undeniable connections among chronic stress, weight gain, and vital sign. Although we can't always control how stressful our lives are, there are certain steps that every and each one among us can fancy better manage the strain we do encounter. Let's take a glance at three unique strategies you'll employ to assist better manage your stress:

Exercise regularly: It should come as no surprise that during a book all about diet and exercise, I'm getting to identify practice as a fundamental stress-management strategy. Even lower-intensity workouts can make an enormous difference in overall health. A recent study published within the journal Health & Place showed that the straightforward act of taking a walk outdoors could help lower your stress levels.

Meditate: Meditation may be a sort of mindfulness that will reap immediate benefits in terms of adjusting the tide of a stressful day. Numerous folks are burdened continuously by all of the items happening in our lives, including our expectations of ourselves and what we face before us in both the short and future.

Secular mindfulness meditation, which may be wiped out a quiet room during a seated position together with your eyes open or closed, is all about naturally breathing while focusing only on the breath and the way your body responds to it. You don't want to regulate the breathing, nor does one want your mind to wander. Start with two to 3 minutes daily— believe me, it's tougher than it sounds.

Need more support or an additional push? Try a meditation smartphone application like Calm, Headspace, and, therefore, the Mindfulness App.

Seek the assistance of friends and family: Share what's on your mind with someone who you trust but who isn't directly associated with what's causing you stress. We frequently underestimate the worth of only getting things off our chests and, therefore, the effects of straightforward pleasures like smiling and laughter in helping us mediate the consequences of a stressful day.

Weight Loss Errors to Avoid

When we consider weight management, our minds often go-to diet and exercise. What's more important than hitting the gym is exercising our brain. If we confirm that the first vital organ in our body is taken care of, we will be sure that other healthy habits will soon follow.

You can diet, exercise, and do everything else you would like to reduce, but if you continually distract, deflect, or hell for leather avoid your problems and root issues, you'll never find true happiness.

The happier you're and, therefore, the more aware you'll be of your psychological state, the higher it'll be within the end, which can also cause an overall better quality of life.

Keep a Journal

Keeping a journey may be a healthy habit for several people regardless of their goals, but it's essential for somebody that desires to reduce also. By writing down your different portion measurements and exercise habits, you'll better make sure that you'll have a basis for evaluation.

When this is often done, you'll predict future problems that may keep you from your goals by looking back on the times of recorded mistakes or slipups. You'll see what sorts of schedules and structures aren't working, so you'll create better habits within the end. The more extensive your journaling, the higher you'll be ready to organize your research study of your weight-loss journey, meaning you'll share your progress or use it as a structure for future diets.

Avoid the Size

The biggest issue with weight-loss strugglers comes once they see the amount on the size. Someone that desires to lose ten pounds might get discouraged if they find they only lost nine. Sometimes, people might even need to gain weight before they find yourself losing a pound. By avoiding the size altogether, individual failures and disappointments are often avoided also.

Find a special thanks for tracking your progress. You'll have monthly weigh-ins, but it shouldn't be something that ought to be checked once each day. Our weight fluctuates such a lot throughout our journey that it isn't worth stressing over on a day today. Any checking that happens quite once each day is additionally likely a nasty habit; you're using it to distract yourself from a much bigger issue.

The Calorie Myth

When many of us diet, they focus an excessive amount of calories. They'll see that a particular snack pack only features a hundred calories, which suggests that it's good for you, right? Wrong. Once we focus an excessive amount of on what percentage calories are in something, we're failing to seem in the least the different factors that structure that product. Something with zero calories might include harmful chemicals or hidden substances that are bad for us. Something with plenty of calories could be avoided, albeit it's an outsized number of vitamins and necessary fiber.

Calories should still be considered, because the more calories you're taking in, the more you've got to burn through exercise. They always shouldn't be a basis for what foods you opt to eat. If you focus an excessive amount of calories, you'll find yourself losing sight of other important issues. Remember that weight loss isn't about numbers. What's on the size or the nutrition package is vital in ensuring measurements, but they shouldn't be the definitive goals that you're creating on your weight-loss journey.

Talk About It

Keeping things in isn't right. It can feel pretty awful. People who are overweight might find themselves feeling embarrassed about their weight. Maybe they find yourself making excuses for themselves once they eat certain foods, verbalizing these reasons to others around them as a sort of validation. "Oh, I'll just start my diet tomorrow," you would possibly hear someone say as they sneak a couple of extra cupcakes from the dessert table. Instead, try talking about the problems and struggles you've got instead of about the way you're getting to structure for your issues later. You would possibly find that you simply find yourself getting some great advice from an individual that's browsing the same struggle.

It's essential to be an honest listener also. Sometimes, people aren't trying to find answers or advice when they're complaining about their issues. It’s nice only to have someone to vent to each once during a while.

Avoid telling people about your goal before you get on target, however. Talking about your feelings, emotions, and struggles is usually an honest thing. Sometimes it just takes saying something aloud for it to feel real. However, many of us set themselves up for failure by sharing their goals too early. People who post on social media about how they’re getting to reduce are less likely to follow through with their goals. Stay silent with the bulk at the start of your journey, confiding in only those you recognize you'll believe and trust.

Binge Eating

Understanding your binge eating habits is vital, as this enables you to develop conscious awareness and a way of mindfulness around why you're binge eating within the first place. Once you are ready to understand why you binge eat, resolving the basis explanation for your binge eating becomes easier because you recognize what to seem for and what to remember.

Getting to the basis explanation for your binge eating is often done by reflecting on your binge eating cycles and, if necessary, tracking your binge eating cycles. So that you'll start to spot any possible patterns that exist around your binge eating behaviors. You'll easily do that by keeping a food diary, which may be a journal where you log everything you've got eaten during a day.

Make sure that you simply write down the time that you ate, what you ate, and the way much you ate. Track everything, including little snacks in between.

They may not seem significant, but you would possibly be surprised to ascertain how they add up and what comes of these snacks. Often, people find that they're unaware of how problematic their snacking has become until they start to trace it.

As you start trying to find the basis explanation for your binge eating, you would possibly find that there are a couple of root causes. Often, however, most binge eating patterns are traced back to at least one “major” root problem that seems to make more problems than the remainder. For instance, you would possibly find that you simply have poor eating habits and sometimes end up craving low-quality food, but you would probably realize that this largely stems from you being an emotional eater.

Or, you would possibly find that you simply are an emotional eater because you've got poor eating problems, then you realize that, during a flash of stress, eating is one thing you'll look out of while everything else might sound out of your control.

It is important that you simply take the time to spot every single root explanation for your binge eating and not just the one that stands out the foremost. If you're getting to have the most critical impact on changing your binge eating patterns, you're getting to get to know everything that contributes to your binge eating so that you'll be mindful of what could be triggering this behavior.

If you are doing not specialize in and heal all of your root causes for binge eating, you would possibly end up binge eating out of habit and justifying it by different root causes every single time.

The more thorough you'll be with healing this, the simpler you'll be, too.

With that being said, you'll find it to be particularly overwhelming to aim to truly resolve all of your root causes directly, especially if you've got a couple of. If it does feel overwhelming, you'll focus instead on just handling the most important one, then healing one root cause at a time.

This way, you'll make a significant impact on healing your binge eating problems, but you're still ready to remain mindful and conscious of your other binge eating triggers.

Learning to Avoid Temptations and Triggers

Once you've got a clear understanding of what your binge eating cycles and patterns are like, you'll start implementing change to assist you to avoid temptations and triggers. There are some ways that you simply can reasonably avoid temptations and triggers when it involves eliminating binge eating; however, you're getting to got to focus even as much on your mindset as you are doing on your behaviors if you would like to really change.

This way is where meditation goes to assist you to begin to start out engaging in proper portion control so that you're not in danger of binge eating anymore.

With meditation and hypnosis, you'll begin to resolve the deep subconscious reasons behind your binge eating behaviors so that you've got a neater time adhering to your changes. The more you engage during this deep healing, the better it's getting to be for you to form conscious and mindful changes in your eating habits, too.

As you employ meditation and hypnosis to assist you to stop binge eating, you furthermore may get to specialize in actually intentionally avoiding temptations and triggers.

There are many practical ways in which you'll mindfully eliminate these temptations and triggers from your life.

For example, you would possibly intentionally stop buying the kinds of foods that you simply regularly binge eat so that the temptation does not exist to start with.

You might also confirm that you simply eat a normal schedule so that you're not fasting to the purpose of being so hungry that you cannot stop yourself. If that's hard for you, learning habits like meal prepping may be a great opportunity for you to stop yourself from waiting too long between meals then binge eating as how to form up for missing out on foods.

Other famous thanks to starting overcoming binge eating are to acknowledge that emotions are often a severe trigger.

In recognizing that, you'll prefer to identify and enlist new coping methods to assist you in navigating emotions during a healthier way that doesn't include binge eating. This way, you're more likely to manage your feelings with proper emotional management tools, instead of trying to numb yourself with the satisfaction that you simply get from snacking on junk foods.

If you discover that anything ex-directory here tends to be a temptation or trigger for you to binge and eat, confirm that you simply remain conscious of it, which you begin offsetting it by changing your habits and behaviors. The more you'll become aware of your patterns and cycles, the better it'll be for you to seek out ways to beat these patterns and sequences so that you'll have a healthier relationship with food.

150 Weight Loss Positive Affirmations

These are all phrases that you simply should tell yourself as often as possible. As we read them, allow them to flow through your mind as if they're your own.

Write the words right down to remember those further, put notes around your house with the affirmations written on them, or just find other creative ways to include these affirmations in your life. Let's start reading them now so that you'll get these ideas in your head directly.

I even have a cheerful and healthy attitude towards life.

I like my body; that's why I would like the simplest for it.

I like myself; that's why I would like to be healthy.

My health is my utmost priority.

My body is wonderful, and that I love myself at the top of the day.

I can feel my body getting slimmer a day.

I can feel my appetite getting more manageable a day.

I think in my capability to succeed in my goals of complete weight loss.

A day I weigh myself, the scales show significant weight loss.

Every day I successfully reduce without fail.

My weight loss program is functioning like magic.

My body is responding immensely to my weight loss efforts.

I can feel my body fat melting away.

I even have developed a high rate of metabolism that helps me reach my ideal weight.

I even have entirely specialized in my weight loss journey.

Once I set a goal, I confirm I achieve it.

A day I awaken challenged and determined to succeed in my ideal weight goal.

Nobody and zip can stop me from stepping into the simplest shape of my life.

My determination to reduce can't be deterred.

My motivation to exercise is outstanding.

A day I'm motivated to follow a daily exercise regimen.

I'm self-motivated and inspired to reduce and follow a healthy lifestyle.

I have already got a transparent picture in my head of how sexy and beautiful/handsome I look once I finally reach my ideal weight.

Being healthy isn't only a life-style on behalf of me but a principle that I'm determined to keep.

I select to be a healthy and fit person.

I select to eat healthily and maintain a lively lifestyle.

I select to feel fit and sexy.

My mind is hard-wired to require only healthy food, and my body automatically feels the need for daily physical activity.

My mind only accepts Positive thoughts and compliments about my body and resists any negativities, which will divert me far away from my weight loss goal.

30 I am surrounded by people that help and motivate me during my weight loss journey.

I feel grateful for my body and the way effectively it responds to my weight loss efforts.

I'm grateful for my reliable will power and skill to manage my weight.

I'm thankful for the people that are helping me reach my final weight loss goals.

I can easily divert myself from restaurants and establishments, which will function as a temptation to practice unhealthy eating habits.

I can easily resist processed food, refined sugars, and salty snacks.

I even have developed a healthy eating habit.

I keep myself hydrated to assist in my weight loss.

I even have established a daily exercise regimen that's very easy on behalf of me to follow.

I even have embraced a lifetime of clean and healthy living.

I even have finally reached my ideal weight.

I'm successful in my goal of total weight loss.

I invite all challenges that cause a greater understanding of myself and my purpose.

My essence guides me daily toward better choices for my body.

I'm blessed by the alternatives I make.

I'm blessed by my ability to settle on.

I even have insights bestowed for my greater good.

I answer those insights wisely and enthusiasm.

I even have used my intuition to develop sound confidence in my decisions.

I'm what I even have continuously thought and acted on.

I'm the transformation the planet needs immediately.

I'm the living embodiment of belief in action.

I exploit my body for exercise, and my mind for belief, and my heart for forgiveness.

I even have an option to be who I would like to be.

Thereupon choice, I select to let the flow of universal knowledge speak through me as a vessel of assertiveness.

I speak back to the universal flow with my actions.

I recognize those needs altogether their usefulness, and that I claim them for the roadmap to my self-appointed weight loss goals.

I'm what I specialize in.

I'm the reality of my focus.

I really like myself with a full heart.

I really like my body with a full heart.

I really like myself with a full mind.

I really like exercising with a full spirit.

I'm the love I want in my life.

64 I am healthy and my ideal weight.

65. I exploit my skills, knowledge, and resources to form the simplest food choices for my life.

66. I shine outward from within, and my body is an example of my inner beauty.

67. I welcome the challenge of exercise.

68. I welcome my sense of private change.

69. I welcome my higher truth to talk through me.

70. I welcome my goals as benchmarks to assist me in achieving my ultimate level of happiness.

71. I boldly conquer all obstacles.

72. I'm thankful to receive these challenges to use my will to persevere.

73. I'm appreciative of the challenges in my life for a way they teach me to succeed.

74. I'm successful because I even have been tested and passed the tests with flying colors.

75. I'm surrounded by teachers that provide me an opportunity to be my greatest self a day.

76. I'm continuously thankful for my mentors, who show me the way to overcome my doubts.

77. I'm grateful for those that know my true worth and challenge me to ascertain it in myself.

78. I move my body to eliminate stress.

79. I gravitate towards healthy decisions.

80. I rest my body after tireless effort.

81. I'm the bravery I like in others.

82. I enter that bravery with a warrior's spirit, ready for the challenges ahead.

83. That truth gives me the facility to form wise choices.

84. I'm the mountain.

85. I'm the climber.

86. I put faith in my tools, for they assist me on my climb.

87. My motivation inspires my climb.

88. My tools assist me in my option to persevere and succeed on my very own.

89. I'm the mountain I even have conquered.

90. I'm a warrior.

91. My spirit is alive with the facility to strike.

92. I'm swift.

93. I'm cunning.

94. I'm an observer peering through a veil of disbelief.

95. Where others see obstacles, I see opportunities.

96. I spring forth and capture my target.

97. I exclaim in victory.

98. I bow in remembrance and respect for my journey.

99 My choices are fertile ground for continued success.

100. I water my aspirations.

101. I fertilize my goals.

102. That created the oceans.

103. The Volcanoes.

104. The minerals.

105. The air.

106. I hail from that which is seen and unseen.

107. I'm the facility of creation.

108. I select to use that power to succeed in my weight loss goals.

109. Today, I claim the healthy fit body that has always been mine.

110. Today, I'm thrilled to receive the facility that I used to be entitled to at birth.

111. I'm here to experience great joys and great triumphs.

112. I'm the force that awakens.

113. I even have the body I also have always wanted.

114. Salvation is mine to behold.

115. Beauty is mine to behold.

116. I'm valued because I think in my ability to be the person I used to be always meant to be.

117. I'm the visionary for the projection of my life.

118. I'm actively viewing and participating and enjoying and creating the flow of my life.

119. I've chosen a healthy life as my expression.

120. I've chosen beauty as my call.

121. I'm changing.

122. Constant change.

123. I count my change in my vault of strength.

124. I overflow with the change, and thus, I'm healthy.

125. My bank is full and bursting at the seams because I dare to vary.

126. I allow the dreams of possibilities to manifest in my lifestyle.

127. I attract the facility of the universe as a welcome addition to assist me in my weight loss goals.

128. Exude positivity.

129. The manifestation of constant evolution envelops me.

130. I'm a phoenix rising out of the flames of yesterday.

131. I'm appreciative of this alteration and consider it as an affirmation of my true destiny.

132. I'm grateful.

133. I would like to urge a slim.

134. I'm appreciative.

135. I'm blessed.

136. I'm happy.

137. I'm loved.

138. I'm proud to precise myself through my exercise.

139. I'm rewarded, hourly, daily, monthly, and yearly for my achievements through my persistent workouts.

140. I'm rewarded for my efforts.

141. I'm fit and healthy.

142. I'm my very own salvation.

143. My attitude determines my success.

144. I achieve my goals with ease because I think.

145. I select to be thin.

146. I'm living my target weight.

147. I'm the healthiest I am often in the least times.

148. I'm empowered.

149. I'm powerful.

150. I'm dedicated.

A 30-Day Challenge

Day 1

Set a weight-loss target

Read your daily affirmation

Set a goal and obtain yourself ready

Meal

A Whole Egg with oatmeal and little Glass of skimmed milk

Day 2

Clean out your fridge

Read your daily affirmation

Dispose of items not good for your body

Cream of Wheat with Glass of skimmed milk

Day 3

Stock up on superfoods

Read your daily affirmation

Get all meals and food ready

Celery Sticks

Day 4

Assess your personality

Read your daily affirmation

Grilled Salmon with Asparagus

Day 5

Find time for fitness

Engage fitness and major bodywork

Push up, walk around,

Read your daily affirmation

Grilled pigeon breast with small sweet potato

Day 6

Cut your portions

Read your daily affirmation.

Apple with ¼ few unsalted almonds

Day 7

Do a strength workout

Read your daily affirmation

Oatmeal with skimmed milk

Day 8

Eat more fat-burning foods

Read your daily affirmation

Peaches with Low-Sugar Yogurt

Day 9

Drop bad workout habits

Read your daily affirmation

Broiled Salmon with tossed salad

Day 10

Toss these low-fat foods

Read your daily affirmation

Sweet Potato with Broiled Turkey Burgers

Day 11

Read your daily affirmation

Do a 15-minute Speed circuit workout Can of Tuna with Watermelon.

Day 12

Read your daily affirmation Eat a high protein breakfast grain bread and spread

Low Fat or skimmed milk

Day 13

Read your daily affirmation

Go vegetarian—for each day

Plain Low-Fat Yogurt used as Dip for Veggie Sticks

Day 14

Read your daily affirmation

Do fat-burning body workout

Baked Tilapia with Cold Spinach Salad

Day 15

Curb post-workout snacking

Read your daily affirmation

Grain Bread and a few Egg Whites

Day 16

Control cravings

Read your daily affirmation

Fiber dry cereal with skimmed milk

Day 17

Sculpt your butt, legs, and core

Read your daily affirmation

A Couple of Low-Fat Cheese Sticks and a Mango

Day 18

Search for hidden sugar

Read your daily affirmation

Grilled Tilapia and Whole Wheat Pasta

Day 19

Skip packaged foods

Read your daily affirmation

1 Cup of Low Sugar Yogurt with Strawberries

Day 20

Slim down your home

Read your daily affirmation

Canned Chicken with a Sliced Cucumber

Day 21

Unleash your inner animal

Read your daily affirmation

Fiber dry cereal with low fat

Day 22

Turn up your metabolism Read your regular affirmation turkey sandwich with low-fat cheese on whole

Day 23

Boost good bacteria

Read your daily affirmation

Unsalted almonds and a little pear

Day 24

Make a couple of servings of quinoa

Read your daily affirmation

Celery Sticks with spread

Day 25

Do ballet-inspired workout

Read your daily affirmation

Chicken Breast, with Grain Bread

Day 26

Weigh yourself

Read your daily affirmation

Lean grilled pork chops w/ green beans

Day 27

Do this jump-rope workout

Read your daily affirmation

Oatmeal with Turkey Bacon small glass of skimmed milk

Day 28

Discover your fifth taste

Read your daily affirmation

Grilled pigeon breast and asparagus

Day 29

Try these plank variations

Read your daily affirmation

Peanut butter and banana sandwich on whole wheat or grain bread

Day 30

Get inspired!

Read your daily affirmation

Walnuts (Unsalted) with an Orange

Weight Loss Tips and Tricks

To achieve your weight loss goals, you want to be willing to let any fear and doubt you'll have about hypnotherapy, go. It's not something that you simply can second guess, particularly not its effectivity and results-driven orientation. It's an answer used for several different reasons, even aside from weight loss. Hypnotherapy for weight loss can assist you in overcoming a negative relationship with food, one which will have formed over a period or throughout your entire life. It's something which will present you with proper results which you'll always be sure of.

Although it's not a diet or weight loss supplement, it fulfills an identical supporting role and is the inspiration on the journey of living a more mindful lifestyle. Since the tactic thereof is concentrated on replacing old negative habits with new positive ones, it helps one to beat challenges faced when trying to reduce.

Whether you would like to choose a one-on-one weight loss for hypnotherapy session or simply hear audiobooks online, both can serve you usefully.

Before you dive into the planet of hypnotherapy, you ought to know that there are tons more to it than you'll have initially thought. Very similar to Yoga and meditation, generally, it serves a greater purpose because it leads you on to a mindful path of physical, mental, and emotional wellness.

Tips for Hypnosis for Weight Loss

Find the proper hypnotherapist for weight loss for you. How would you set about doing this, you'll ask? Rather than going the obvious route of checking out hypnotherapists online in your area, why not invite recommendations instead? Honestly, what's better than asking a lover, loved one, or acquaintance to recommend you an honest hypnotherapist for weight loss? If nobody you recognize knows a hypnotherapist that's known for the outstanding jobs they perform, then you'll want to see together with your doctor and invite advice. They ought to be ready to recommend a professional and results-oriented hypnotherapist for weight loss. To make sure you've got the proper hypnotherapist, make certain to see with yourself whether their consultation felt as if it had been thorough. Know if the hypnotherapy program is adjusted to satisfy your needs and also if the practitioner helped answer your questions. Once they leave space between sessions, it shows you're handling an honest hypnotherapist.

Don't Pay Any Attention to Advertising

We sleep in 2020, which suggests that everything we see online is taken seriously. However, it should not be. People are oblivious and vulnerable to accept everything they read or hear, but when it involves advertising, not everything is often trusted. Advertising should, ever often, be disregarded and not taken too seriously because it is often very misleading. It is usually better to conduct your research before you merely accept that something may be a certain way or not. Within the case of hypnotherapy, since there are numerous negative associations associated with the practice, it is best to seek out what's it all about yourself. As you'll see from this handy set of data provided about hypnotherapy for weight loss, it's completely safe and doubtless nothing negative that you simply expected it to be.

Get Information About Training, Qualifications, And Necessary Experience

Before you choose a hypnotherapist, you want to make sure about their necessary information first. You want to know: Do they run the practices together or operate independently? Are they certified and have a license? Ensuring that they also adhere to moral standards, most preferably recommended by other medical physicians, you will be assured that you simply are handling someone who knows what they're doing.

Before Choosing One Hypnotherapist, Ask Several First

One of the simplest ways to seek out whether a hypnotherapist is best fitted to you is to speak with a couple of them over a call first. This way may take some effort, but it'll be worthwhile within the end. You've got to think about whether or not they can relate to you, care about your wellbeing, and hear your concerns, whether or not they are personable, accommodating, and professional. If they tick all the boxes, then you're good to travel.

Don't Fall for Any Unrealistic Promises

If a hypnotist tells you that their therapy session will assist you in reducing fast, then don't even bother getting to one session. Hypnosis for weight loss may be a process that takes time. It can take anywhere between three weeks, up to 3 months, to ascertain your human body change and to reduce. Since your body and mind should first adjust, you would like to permit time for it to try to so. Hypnosis for weight loss isn't a fad; neither is it a way of losing weight overnight. It is also essential to avoid hypnotherapists who suggest they're going to cause you to reduce. Since they're going only to be talking during the session, what they're telling you isn't true whatsoever. What you'll expect from a knowledgeable and authentic hypnotherapist, however, maybe a professional individual who takes responsibility for helping you to urge where you would like to travel. This person should assist you in accessing your subconscious with ease and assist you in bringing it on board with a correct weight loss plan and possibly an exercise routine.

Is Your Hypnotherapist of Choice Multi-Skilled?

Even though hypnosis may be a terrific tool and may alter the mind's way of brooding about food, it goes hand-in-hand with nutrition. This way is often something you would like to think about, mainly whether your hypnotist features a good understanding of what it takes for you to reduce sustainably and healthily. Many of us focused on starting a weight loss journey don't necessarily know what they ought to do or what they ought to eat. When trying to find a hypnotherapist, search for one that features a self-help coaching or some sort of psychotherapy qualification, also as a qualification/background in either nutrition or cognitive behavioral therapy.

Find Out the Time You Ought to Engage During A Program

This therapy is quite important as hypnotherapy can become quite expensive if you are going to knowledgeable for one-on-one sessions. If you favor getting to knowledgeable instead of conducting the courses at your home, you'll prefer to spread your sessions out over time to form it cheaper. Albeit you'll think that the sessions subsided effective in achieving the general effect, it works more effectively as your mind and body require time to regulate. Time is additionally required as you modify your old habits and replace them with new ones to reduce.

Questions to Ask

- Ask your hypnotherapist if they will provide you with a program to take care of your progress reception. A recording mainly helps to permit you to opened up sessions over time. Taking note of your weight loss hypnosis recording a day will keep you in restraint and assist you to stay motivated and focused.

As your hypnotherapist, if they will tailor-make your hypnotherapy weight loss program for you. If the therapist complies with it, you'll expect a weight loss hypnotherapy program that's far more effective than individualized hypnosis, offering treatments that will work better than ones that cater to everyone. Since everyone is different compared to others, this makes tons more sense. Sure, the overall program will work, but a customized one could provide you with better results.

- Ask whether your program includes an introduction session. Starting with hypnotherapy for weight loss, you do not want to only dive right into it. It is vital to require the required time, albeit it's just an hour, to determine your needs and concerns regarding your current habits, lifestyle, and goals together with your hypnotherapist. Ensuring that they care about your wellbeing and results rather than just taking you thru the session is equally important. Taking the time to speak to your therapist and going to know them better will assist you to feel more comfortable and form a foundation of trust before starting together with your hypnotherapy sessions.

Establish the prices involved before starting together with your sessions.

Ensuring you recognize what proportion an initial consultation and every session cost are going to be another important factor you've got to think about before choosing a hypnotherapist. Considering the worth, a summary of the therapist program compared to other potential weight loss programs. Review supported the standard of service you'll receive, and take under consideration that you simply can spread your practice over weeks rather than getting to a couple of sessions every week.

Lastly, you ought to view hypnotherapy as an investment in yourself and wellbeing, instead of an unnecessary expense. The context for this thought will realize once you engage in or complete your program.

Tips for Managing Stress to Avoid Emotional Eating

No matter what your binge eating cycles are like, stress is nearly bound to encourage you to interact in emotional eating. When it involves stress and its ability to influence your dietary behaviors, there are generally two ways in which it can happen.

The first is that you simply end up feeling stressed, and you binge eat as how to make some sort of comfort in your life so that you're not feeling quite as stressed anymore. The opposite way includes you feeling so stressed that you simply think that you cannot eat, then binge eating when your body cannot take the stress-induced fasting anymore. In either scenario, stress can negatively affect your diet and may also become a negative coping method that worsens your binge eating within the future, too. Furthermore, both of those behavioral patterns around stress and eating can cause weight gain, which suggests that they're not productive to your goals of weight loss.

Managing stress to avoid emotional eating largely revolves around you learning the way to deal with and manage your stress properly. The more proactive you'll be in handling your pressure, the less likely you're to hunt out behaviors like binge eating as a chance to assist you to overcome the strain that you simply are experiencing.

People who routinely experience problematic binge eating, thanks to stress or other emotions, will often address healthier practices like meditating, preventative self-care, and routine relaxation practices to assist them in reducing stress. This way, they're less likely to interact in emotional eating within the first place.

When it involves handling bursts of upper-stress levels, meditating is often incredibly helpful in assisting you with bringing your stress levels to backtrack. This way, you're more likely to feel asleep and less susceptible to feel the necessity to affect your stress through less healthy means, like through overeating.

Preventative self-care measures that will assist you in affecting your stress are incredibly useful in avoiding stress within the first place. For instance, budgeting more effectively so that you're not so worried about money, creating a bank account, exercising daily, and spending time with loved ones are all great ways to avoid scenarios where your stress may rise unnecessarily.

The simpler you're at handling areas of your life that typically end in stress, the simpler you'll be in eliminating your stress. Or, when it can't be removed, a minimum of minimizing it so that you'll feel more asleep in your life.

Routine relaxation practices are almost like preventative self-care, except that they're more focused on the day to day practices that are meant to assist you to relax regardless of what has triggered your stress.

For example, some people click after work a day and luxuriate in a while gardening, reading a book, or just resting on the couch with their eyes closed so that they need time to decompress from the day they need had. People wish to take a candlelit bath, choose a walk, or maybe play a game on their laptop as how to destress. The thought here is that you simply find a good thanks to decompressing whenever you are feeling stressed, which you are doing it on a day to day in order that your stress doesn't begin to rise an excessive amount of within the first place.

When it involves managing your stress to avoid overeating, the simplest thing you'll do is still try new routines and rituals until you discover practices that assist you in destressing without overeating.

The exact “formula” for destressing is going to be different for everybody, so you're getting to need to take a while to seek out that information out for yourself. The higher you understand your own needs around stress and the way to relax, the more likely you're to be ready to come up with a practice that's getting to assist you in destressing in the first place.

Conclusion

Thank you for creating it through to the end of ***Rapid Weight Loss Hypnosis and Meditation for women***.

This book may be a blend of all the effective techniques to assist people that are affected by excessive weight gain. It presents a special dimension of how the key to weight loss lies in your brain. It covers the techniques of self-hypnosis, Cognitive behavioral therapy (CBT), Sleep Learning, and Meditation. All of those techniques request active involvement of the brain and alter within the wiring pattern of the mind. In this way, it is possible to boost a satisfactory level of the brain to prevent the urges of overeating. The book contains an in-depth account of all the activities, processes, and requirements to form of these techniques healthily compute for you.

This book serves multiple purposes. It not only guides about weight loss techniques but also the basis causes of the opposite emotional problems that promote overeating. This book is a complete guide to a fatless, healthy, happy, and satisfactory lifestyle.

www.ingramcontent.com/pod-product-compliance
Ingram Content Group UK Ltd.
Pitfield, Milton Keynes, MK11 3LW, UK
UKHW020143250726
13967UKWH00002B/832

9 781953 732675